Exercises in Chest X-ray Diagnosis

John A. Elliott BSc, MB, ChB, MRCP
Consultant Physician, with special interest in respiratory diseases,
Heathfield Hospital, Ayr, UK

and

Michael D. Cowan MB, ChB, MRCP, DMRD, FRCR
Consultant Radiologist, Western Infirmary and Knightwood Hospital,
Glasgow, UK

Butterworths
London Boston Durban Singapore Sydney Toronto Wellington

First published, 1987

© Butterworth & Co. (Publishers) Ltd, 1987

British Library Cataloguing in Publication Data

Elliott, John A.
　Exercises in chest X-ray diagnosis.
　1. Chest—Diseases—Diagnosis—
　Problems, exercises, etc.　2. Chest—
　Radiography—Problems, exercises, etc.
　I. Title　II. Cowan, Michael D.
　617'.5407572'076　　　RC941

　ISBN 0-407-00490-4

Library of Congress Cataloging-in-Publication Data

Elliott, John A.
　Exercises in chest X-ray diagnosis.

　Includes bibliographies and index.
　1. Chest—Radiography—Examinations, questions,
etc.　2. Chest—Diseases—Diagnosis—Examinations,
questions, etc.　I. Cowan, Michael D.　II. Title.
[DNLM: 1. Thoracic Radiography—examination questions.
WF 18 E46e]
RC941.E37　1987　　　617'.5407572　　　86-18792
ISBN 0-407-00490-4

Photoset by Butterworths Litho Preparation Department
Printed and bound in England at the University Press, Cambridge

Preface

The chest X-ray is probably the single most common radiographic examination. Its importance as an investigative tool is probably nowhere more evident than in thoracic medicine where an assessment of the standard chest radiograph is usually carried out in parallel with history taking and, for thoracic problems, the chest X-ray might be regarded as an extension of the physical examination. Abnormalities on the chest film may of course reflect purely local thoracic disorders, but may also mirror systemic disease processes. The accurate interpretation of the chest radiograph is a skill that is relevant therefore to all clinicians.

The book is aimed specifically at physicians and radiologists in training. It has been devised principally as a teaching aid for postgraduates working towards the MRCP and FRCP. It provides a test of clinical competence and knowledge, and for this reason a simple question and answer format has been adopted. In such a short book the answer sections are necessarily somewhat limited in scope, providing relatively brief clinical reviews and short accounts of radiological differential diagnosis. In most cases, therefore, key references have been appended to the text throughout. Although the book is obviously intended as an exercise in self assessment, we hope nevertheless to have fulfilled at least in part our broader aim — that of providing readers with the means by which they might improve their skills in chest X-ray interpretation.

Acknowledgements

This book owes much to the enthusiasm of successive cohorts of MRCP and FRCR candidates for whom we have found the contained radiographs a rich source of teaching material. Valuable contributions to our own selection of films have been made by Dr A. Gregor of the Glasgow Institute of Radiotherapeutics and Oncology, Dr R. Monie of the Southern General Hospital, Glasgow, Dr J. McClure of Seafield Children's Hospital, Ayr, Dr F. G. Adams and Dr S. McKechnie, Department of Radiology, Western Infirmary, Glasgow. We are most grateful to Dr R Corbett of the Department of Radiology, Hairmyres Hospital for providing the computed tomography illustrations. Special thanks are due also to Mrs C. Gibson for the customary diligence of her secretarial help and to Mr E. McNulty and Ms V. Preston for their skill and patience in preparing the photographic material upon which the book is based.

Contents

Part 1
Questions

Questions—Plate 1

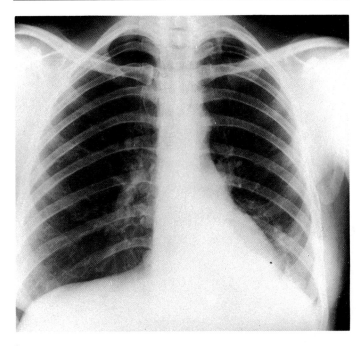

a

This 56-year-old non-smoker with longstanding bronchial asthma gave a two-week history of increased breathlessness and cough productive of tenacious mucoid sputum.

1.1 What is the radiological diagnosis?
1.2 What is the most likely cause in this patient?

Questions—Plate 2

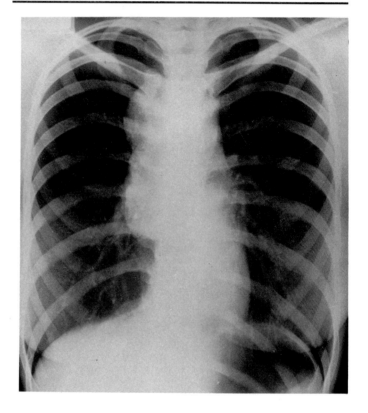

a

Postero-anterior (Plate 2a) and left lateral (Plate 2b) chest radiographs of a 32-year-old woman with dysphagia and generalized muscle weakness of recent onset.

2.1 What is the most likely cause of the radiographic abnormality?

2.2 What is the clinical diagnosis?

4

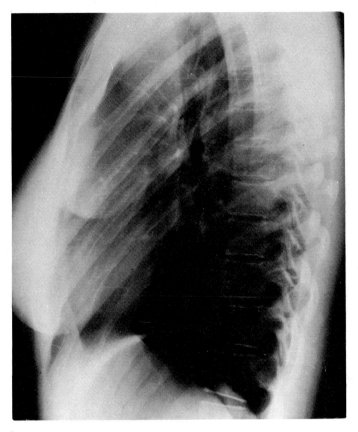

b

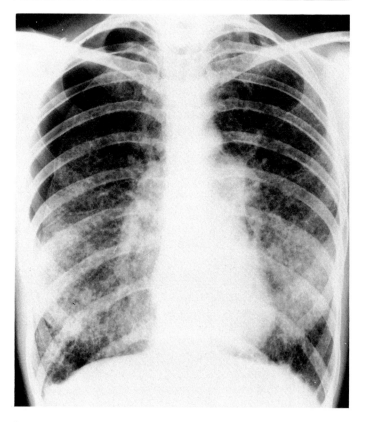

a

For two years this 24-year-old patient complained of progressive breathlessness on exertion before presenting with chest pain associated with a sudden increase of dyspnoea and a short history of thirst and polyuria.

3.1 Give two radiographic abnormalities.
3.2 What is the clinical diagnosis?

Questions—Plate 4

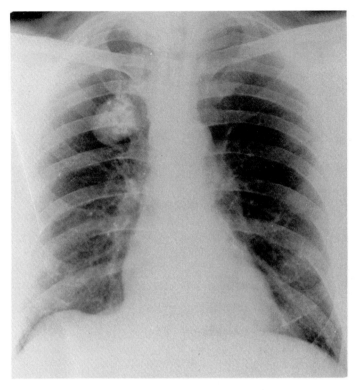

a

This asymptomatic 40-year-old patient was X-rayed for insurance purposes.

4.1 What is the radiological diagnosis?

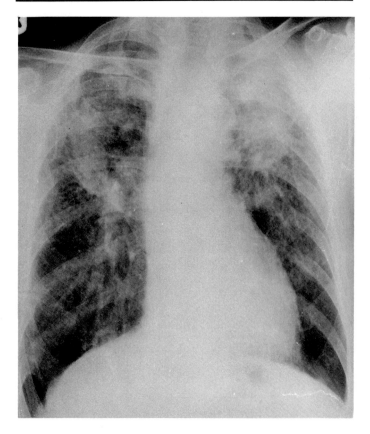

Postero-anterior chest radiograph of a 60-year-old miner with progressive breathlessness and a history of melanoptysis.

5.1 What two radiographic abnormalities are present?
5.2 What are the clinical diagnoses?

Questions—Plate 6

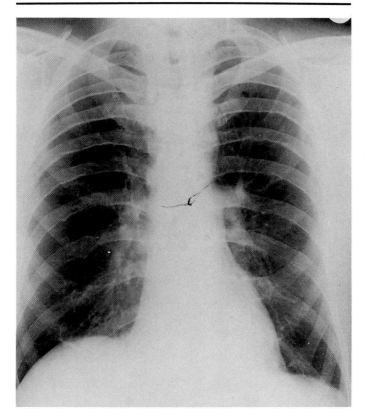

a

This 24-year-old asymptomatic male patient was found to have sustained arterial hypertension.

6.1 What abnormality is shown on this postero-anterior chest radiograph and what is its likely cause in this patient?

6.2 Give three complications of this disorder.

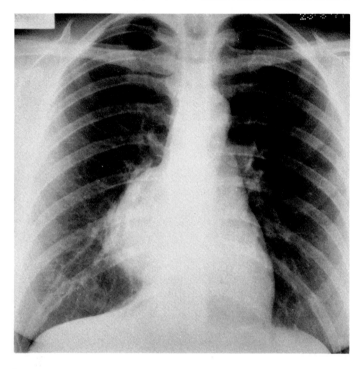

a

Postero-anterior (Plate 7a) and right lateral (Plate 7b) chest radiographs of a 28-year-old asymptomatic female non-smoker referred for investigation following a routine medical examination.

7.1 What is the most likely cause of the radiographic abnormality?

7.2 What two major complications may arise?

Questions—Plate 7

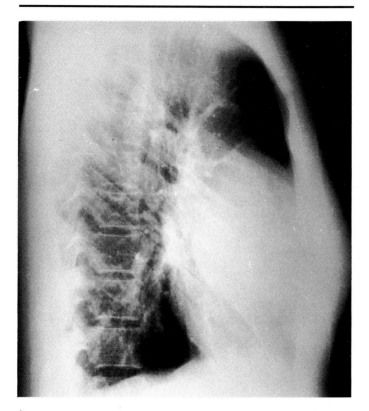

b

11

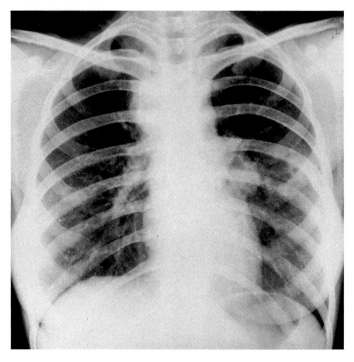

a

This 12-year-old girl was X-rayed as part of a screening programme.

8.1 What are the abnormalities in this postero-anterior radiograph?

8.2 What is the probable clinical diagnosis?

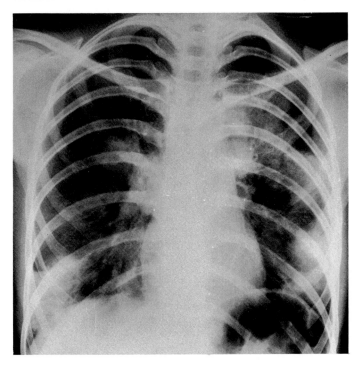

This 30-year-old woman presented with a chronic purulent nasal discharge, normochromic normocytic anaemia and a high ESR.

9.1 What is the most likely clinical diagnosis?

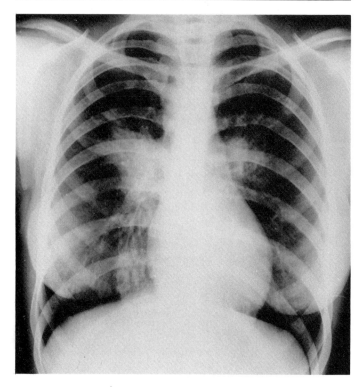

a

This 18-year-old patient with longstanding 'extrinsic' asthma presented with febrile symptoms and cough productive of sputum 'plugs'. Her postero-anterior chest radiographs are shown at presentation (Plate 10a) and ten days later (Plate 10b).

10.1 What clinical entity is likely to be present?
10.2 Suggest three clinical investigations that might help to confirm this diagnosis.

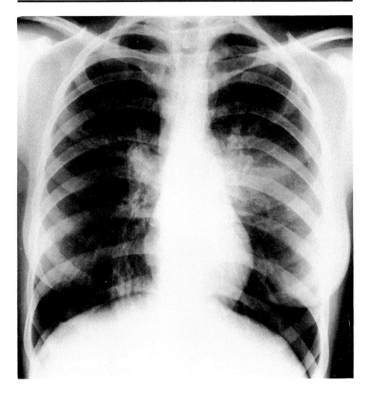

b

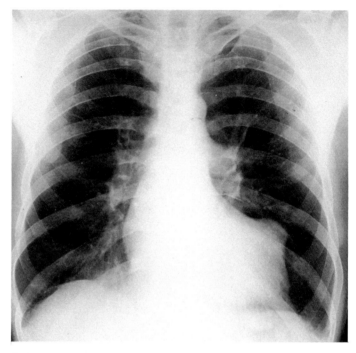

a

Postero-anterior chest radiograph of a 56-year-old man with recurrent syncope.

11.1 What is the radiological diagnosis?
11.2 Give three alternative presentations of this disorder.

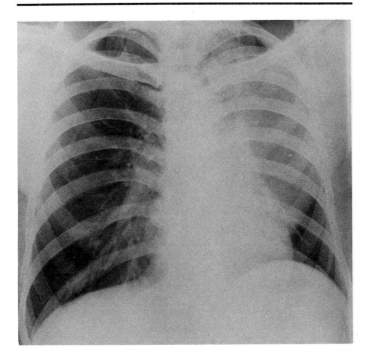

a

Postero-anterior chest radiograph of a 28-year-old non-asthmatic, non-smoker with a five-year history of recurrent left-sided 'pleurisy'.

12.1 What is the radiological diagnosis?
12.2 Suggest the likely clinical diagnosis in this patient.

Questions—Plate 13

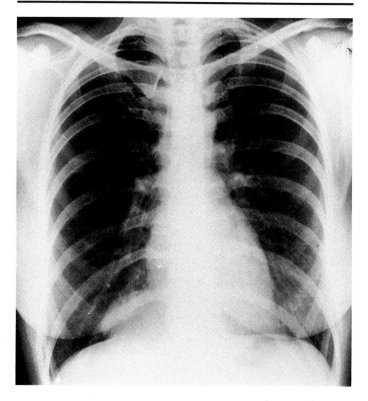

a

Postero-anterior (Plate 13a) and right lateral (Plate 13b) chest radiographs of a 30-year-old asymptomatic non-smoker.

13.1 What is the most likely cause of the radiographic abnormality?

Questions—Plate 13

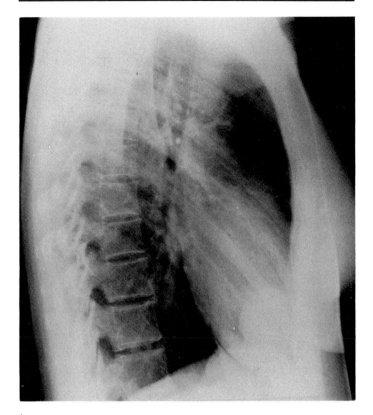

b

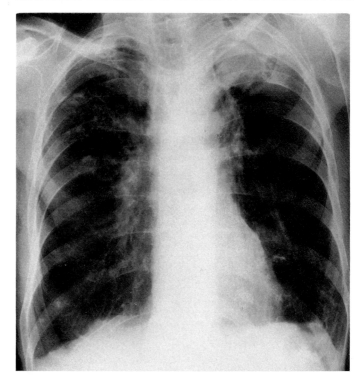

a

This 64-year-old smoker presented with a history of recurrent haemoptysis.

14.1 Give four abnormalities present on the postero-anterior chest radiograph.

14.2 Suggest four relevant investigations.

Questions—Plate 15

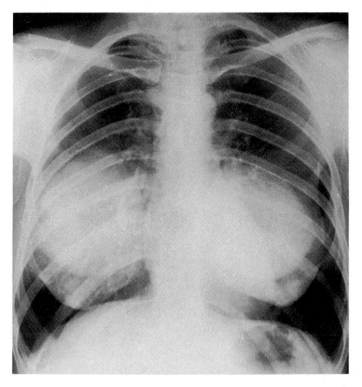

a

This asymptomatic woman was X-rayed for insurance purposes.

15.1 What is the explanation for the bilateral radiographic abnormality?

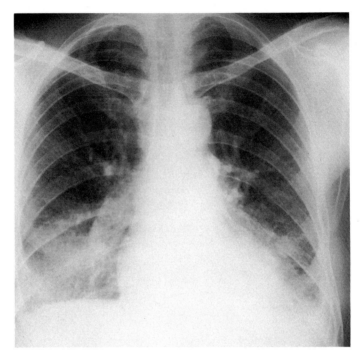

Postero-anterior chest radiograph of a 60-year-old engineering worker with a five-year history of progressive effort dyspnoea.

16.1 What is the most likely clinical diagnosis?
16.2 Suggest two clinical signs that should be sought.

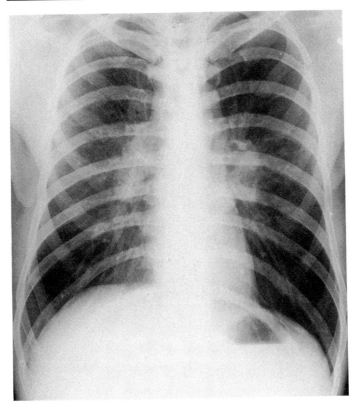

17.1 What abnormality is shown on the postero-anterior chest radiograph?

17.2 Suggest a radiological differential diagnosis.

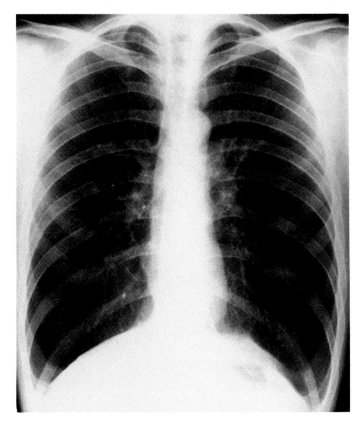

a

18.1 What pathological diagnosis might be inferred from the radiographic appearances in Plates 18*a* and 18*b*?

18.2 The 30-year-old patient whose film is illustrated in Plate 18*a* gave a strong family history of progressive respiratory disease. What clinical entity does this suggest?

Questions—Plate 18

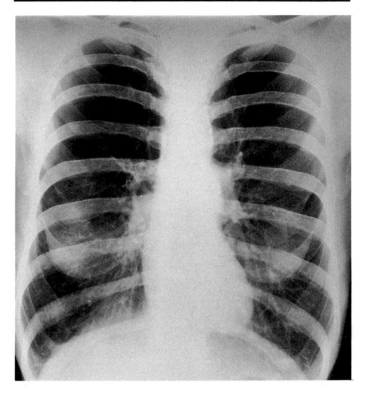

b

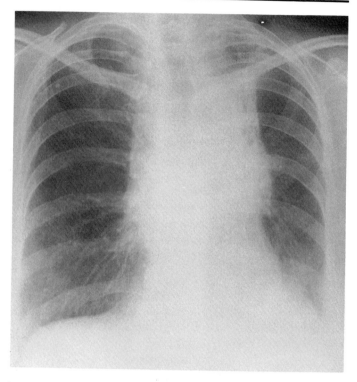

a

This 50-year-old patient complained of a non-productive cough and progressive breathlessness.

19.1 Suggest the most likely cause of the abnormal radiographic appearance in this postero-anterior film.

Questions—Plate 20

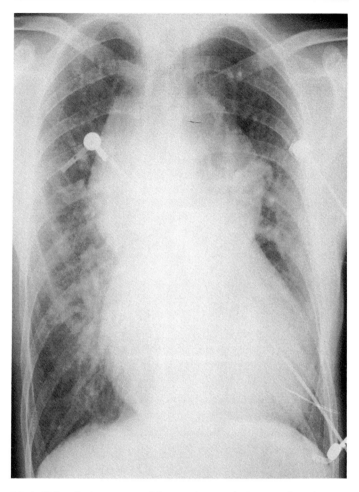

20.1 What is the cause of the mediastinal abnormality shown on this antero-posterior chest film?

20.2 With what cardiac lesion is this condition invariably associated?

Questions—Plate 21

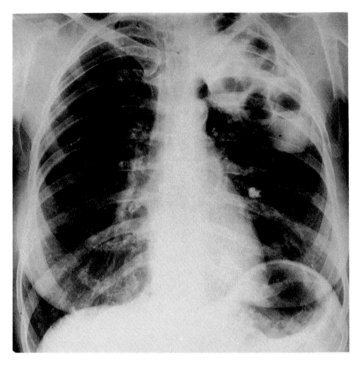

a

This patient gave a history of previous pulmonary tuberculosis.

21.1 What is the explanation for the appearance of the left hemithorax?

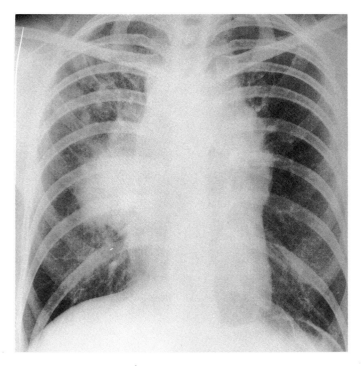

Postero-anterior chest radiograph of a 26-year-old patient presenting with painless cervical lymphadenopathy.

22.1 What is the most likely radiological diagnosis?
22.2 Of which clinical entity is this radiographic appearance particularly suggestive in a young woman?

Questions—Plate 23

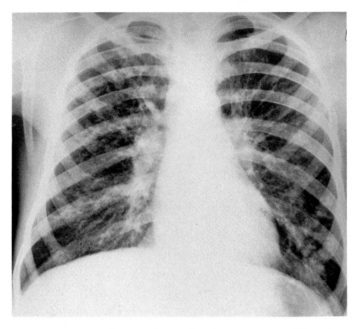

Postero-anterior chest radiograph of an 18-year-old patient with a history of chronic expectoration and recurrent abdominal pain.

23.1 What radiographic abnormalities are present?
23.2 What is the likely clinical diagnosis?
23.3 Suggest the likely cause of the patient's abdominal pain.

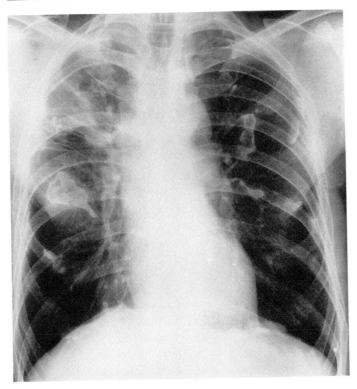

This 60-year-old shipyard worker presented with haemoptysis.

24.1 Give three radiographic abnormalities on the posteroanterior film.

24.2 How might these be related?

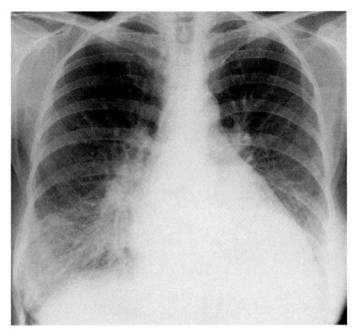

a

25.1 Describe three radiographic abnormalities on this postero-anterior chest film and suggest the radiological diagnosis.

Questions—Plate 26

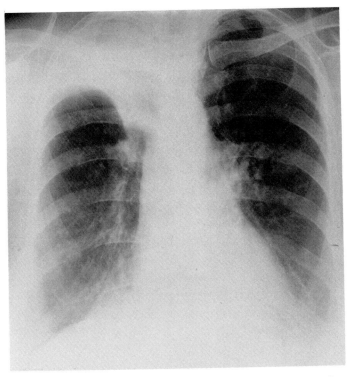

26.1 What radiographic abnormality is illustrated in this postero-anterior chest film?

Questions—Plate 27

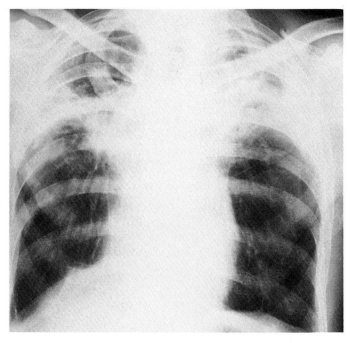

a

This 45-year-old rheumatology outpatient denied any respiratory symptoms.

27.1 What are the two principal radiographic abnormalities seen on the postero-anterior (Plate 27a) and lateral (Plate 27b) chest radiographs?
27.2 What is the underlying clinical diagnosis?

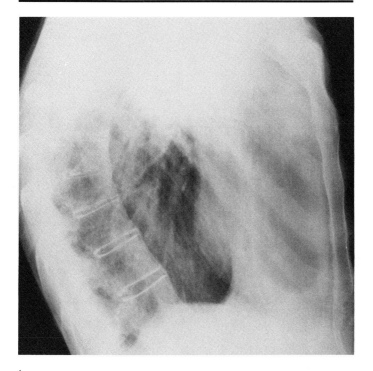

b

Questions—Plate 28

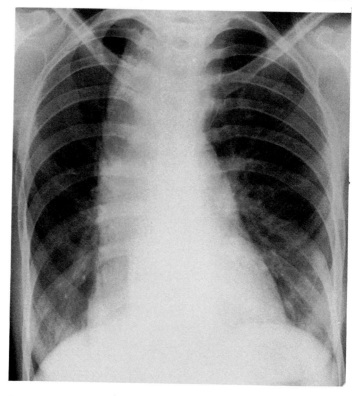

a

This 46-year-old woman gave a history of longstanding dysphagia.

28.1 What is the radiological diagnosis?
28.2 Give three complications of the disorder.

Questions—Plate 29

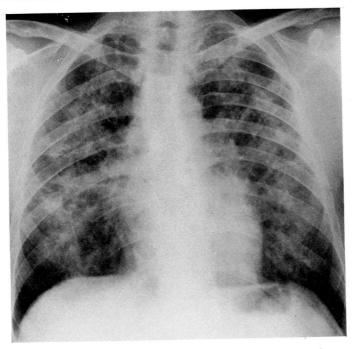

This 46-year-old patient with progressive dyspnoea was also a regular attender at the skin clinic.

29.1 What is the likely radiological diagnosis?

Questions—Plate 30

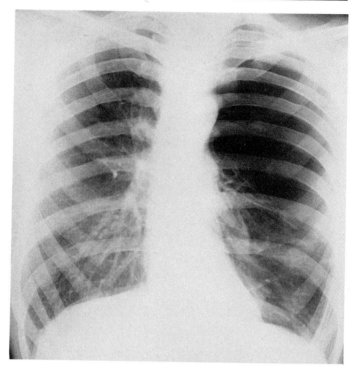

Postero-anterior chest radiograph of a middle-aged smoker.

30.1 What is the radiological diagnosis?
30.2 What are the major clinical features favouring a surgical treatment approach?

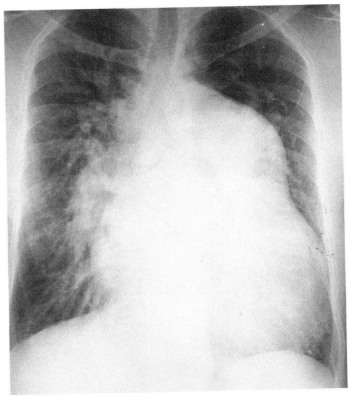

Postero-anterior chest radiograph of a 30-year-old patient with progressive effort dyspnoea and central cyanosis of recent onset.

31.1 Give three radiographic abnormalities.
31.2 What sequence of events best explains the clinical and radiographic features?

Questions—Plate 32

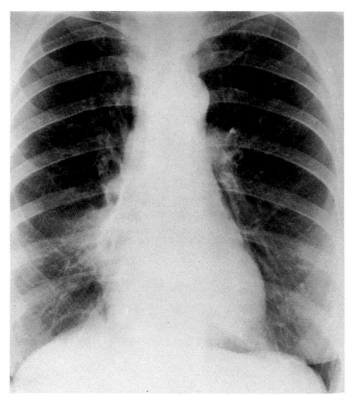

a

Postero-anterior chest radiograph of an elderly smoker with weight loss and haemoptysis.

32.1 What radiographic abnormality is illustrated?

Questions—Plate 33

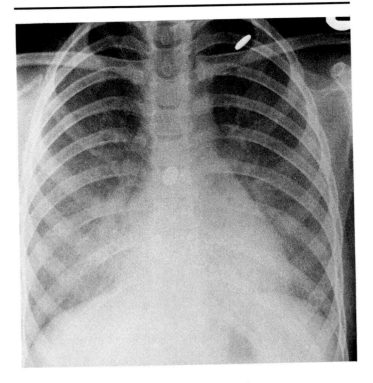

a

This seven-year-old developed an unproductive cough and breathlessness during maintenance treatment for acute leukaemia.

33.1 What is the radiographic abnormality shown on the postero-anterior chest film?

33.2 Suggest a radiological differential diagnosis.

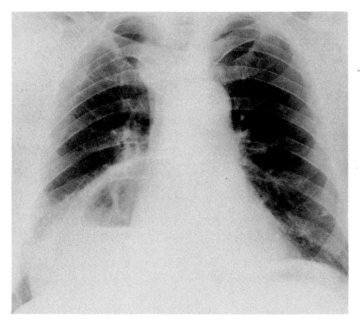

a

Postero-anterior (Plate 34a) and right lateral (Plate 34b) chest radiographs of an elderly asymptomatic patient.

34.1 What is the likely cause of the radiographic abnormality?

34.2 How might this diagnosis be confirmed?

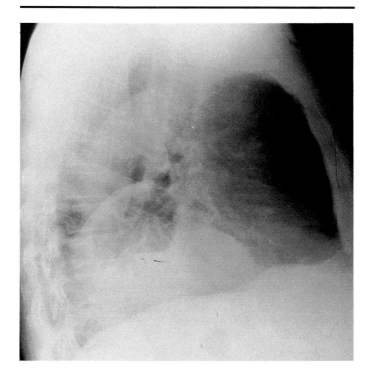

b

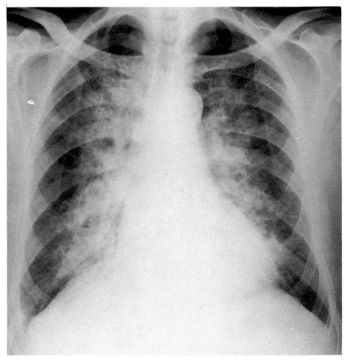

This elderly patient presented with acute breathlessness.

35.1 What is the radiological diagnosis?

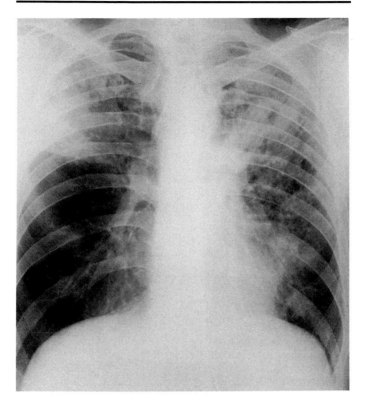

a

Postero-anterior chest radiograph of a 40-year-old patient wth a three-months' history of productive cough and weight loss.

36.1 Describe the radiographic abnormalities.
36.2 What is the most likely clinical diagnosis?

Questions—Plate 37

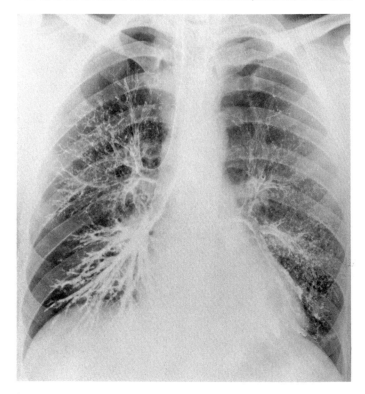

a

Plates 37a and b show postero-anterior and left lateral projections during bilateral bronchography in a 36-year-old patient.

37.1 What is the radiological diagnosis?
37.2 Suggest alternative indications for this investigation.

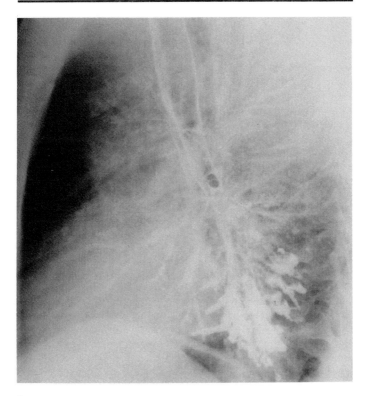

b

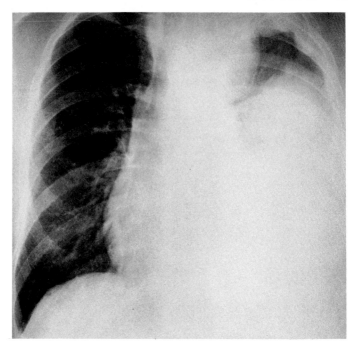

a

Postero-anterior chest radiograph of a 66-year-old retired heating engineer presenting with left-sided chest pain.

38.1 Suggest the likely clinical diagnosis?

Questions—Plate 39

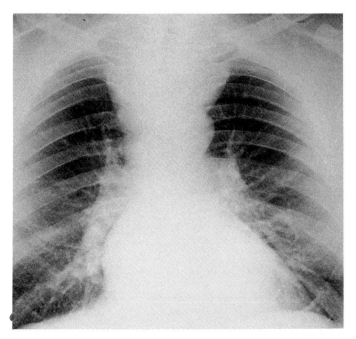

This 56-year-old patient gave a two-year history of progressive effort dyspnoea. Physical examination revealed inspiratory stridor and signs of superior vena caval compression.

39.1 What is the most likely cause of the radiographic abnormality on this postero-anterior film?
39.2 What non-invasive investigation might help confirm this diagnosis?

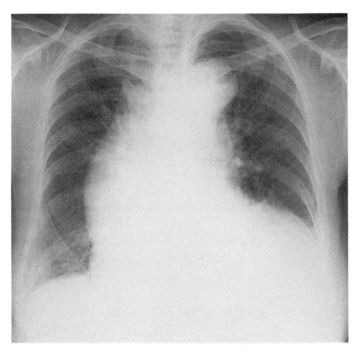

a

This middle-aged man complained of severe central chest pain of sudden onset.

40.1 Describe three abnormalities on the postero-anterior chest radiograph.

40.2 Suggest the likely clinical diagnosis.

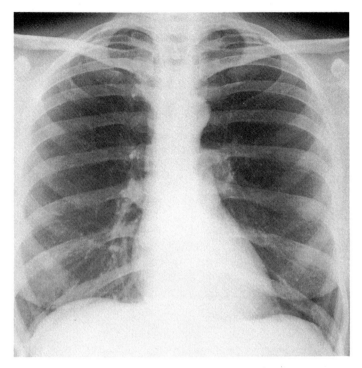

a

Postero-anterior chest radiograph of an asymptomatic adult female. Five years before she had suffered an acute febrile illness associated with a vesicular rash.

41.1 What is the radiographic abnormality?
41.2 What is the clinical diagnosis?

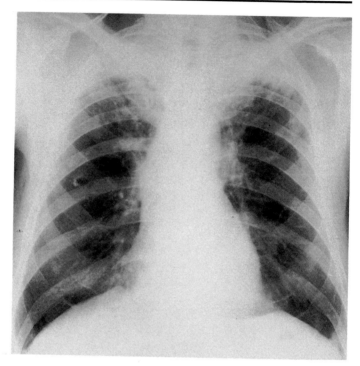

This 63-year-old man presented with a two-month history of febrile symptoms, cough and weight loss. Sputum examination was repeatedly negative for tubercle bacilli. There was a moderate peripheral blood eosinophilia.

42.1 Describe the radiographic abnormality on the postero-anterior film.

42.2 What is the most likely clinical diagnosis?

Questions—Plate 43

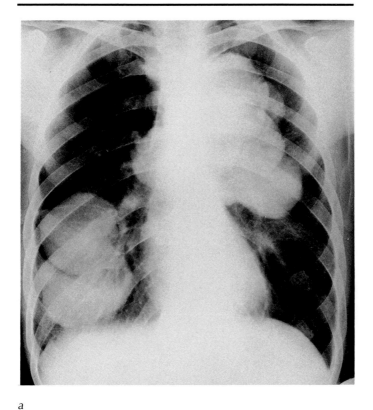

a

43.1 What is the most likely cause of the radiographic abnormality illustrated by this postero-anterior film?

43.2 Give three alternative causes of multiple large circular homogeneous shadows.

Questions—Plate 44

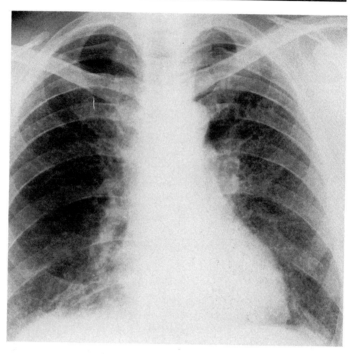

a

Postero-anterior chest radiograph (Plate 44a) and barium swallow (Plate 44b) of a middle-aged woman with progressive breathlessness.

44.1 What are the two most significant radiographic abnormalities?

44.2 Suggest the likely clinical diagnosis.

Questions—Plate 44

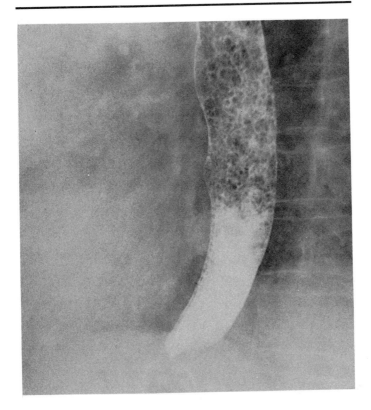

b

55

Questions—Plate 45

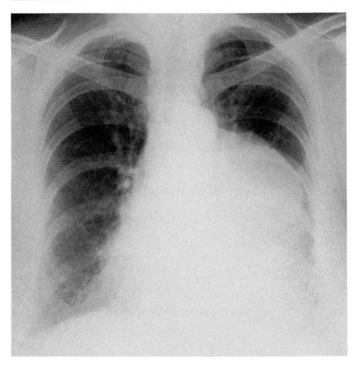

a

Postero-anterior (Plate 45a) chest radiograph of an asymptomatic 70-year-old woman. Plate 45b shows the corresponding thoracic computed tomograph (CT) scan at the level of the aortic arch.

45.1 What is the CT abnormality?
45.2 Suggest a radiological differential diagnosis given that the patient's chest radiograph 20 years earlier had shown a similar appearance.

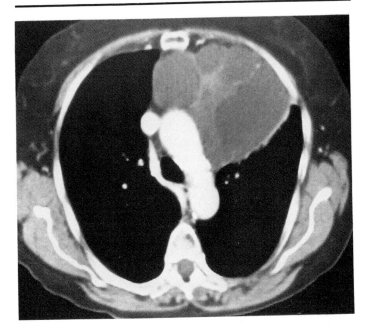

b

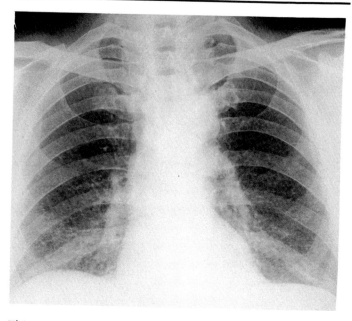

This 56-year-old boiler scaler was X-rayed for insurance purposes.

46.1 What is the radiographic abnormality and what is the likely cause in this patient?

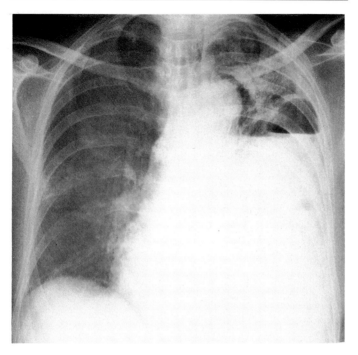

a

This elderly patient with a long history of benign peptic oesophagitis became acutely ill following elective hospital treatment.

47.1 Give two radiographic abnormalities visible on the antero-posterior chest film.

47.2 Suggest the most likely explanation for these appearances in this patient.

Questions—Plate 48

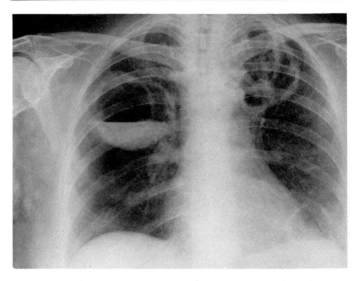

48.1 Describe three radiographic abnormalities in this postero-anterior film.

48.2 Suggest the likely clinical diagnosis.

Questions—Plate 49

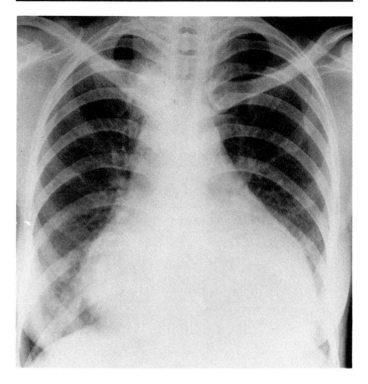

a

Postero-anterior chest radiograph of a 42-year-old woman with systemic lupus erythematosus.

49.1 Suggest the most likely cause of the radiographic abnormality.

49.2 How might this be confirmed non-invasively?

Questions—Plate 50

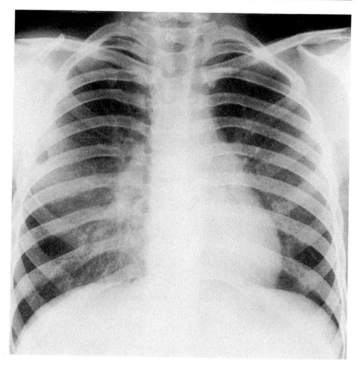

Following an afternoon sojourn in Trafalgar Square this young tourist became unwell after her evening meal with an unproductive cough and increasing breathlessness.

50.1 What radiographic abnormality is shown on the postero-anterior chest film?

50.2 What is the likely clinical diagnosis?

50.3 Suggest three relevant investigations.

Part 2
Answers

Answers—Plate 1

1.1 Left lower-lobe collapse.

1.2 Mucus plugging.

Each pulmonary lobe collapses in a characteristic way. Plate 1a shows the classical appearances of left lower-lobe collapse: there is a triangular shaped homogeneous opacity superimposed on the cardiac shadow, obliterating the medial portion of the left leaf of the diaphragm. This represents the shrunken, airless left lower lobe. In addition, the left hilum has been displaced downwards and is almost invisible. The cardiac shadow is displaced to the left so that the right hilum and right vertebral border are more clearly defined than usual. Plate 1b shows the corresponding appearances produced by collapse of the right lower lobe.

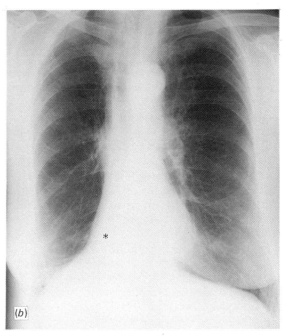

(b)

Plate 1b   Right lower lobe collapse due to mucus impaction in a 50-year-old chronic bronchitic: asterisk denotes triangular shadow of airless lobe at cardiophrenic angle; small hilar vessels; distinct right heart border.

65

Table 1 Radiological signs of lobar collapse

Loss of radiographic lung volume
Reduction in number of pulmonary vessels
Presence of a radio-opacity
Absence of an air bronchogram
Compensatory overinflation
Displacement of landmarks
 – hilar shadows
 – fissures
 – mediastinum
 – diaphragm
Approximation of ribs

The radiological signs of lobar collapse are as listed in Table 1. Loss of volume in the affected hemithorax is usually a major feature and is clearly evident in the example shown in Plate 1a. Complete collapse of a lobe, without associated consolidation, usually produces a detectable opacity on the chest radiograph. Partial collapse produces little opacification unless accompanied by an element of consolidation. Because the airways distal to an obstructed bronchus are usually fluid-filled an air bronchogram cannot be made out within the area of opacity. This contrasts with the appearances in lobar pneumonia when abnormal radiographic shadowing is associated with patent major airways and an air bronchogram can usually be seen. When elements of collapse and consolidation are present simultaneously, loss of volume may be relatively slight and anatomical displacement of neighbouring structures correspondingly less. Significant loss of volume frequently results in compensatory over-inflation of the unaffected lobe(s), as a result of which the remaining pulmonary vessels, which are reduced in number, are more sparsely distributed than normal.

Displacement of a fissure constitutes one of the most important features of collapse and will be referred to again in later examples. Mediastinal displacement is variable occurring most commonly in younger patients and in association with collapse of one of the larger lobes, especially the left upper lobe. Upward diaphragmatic displacement is also variable and is frequently absent, particularly with upper-lobe collapse. Hilar displacement may be marked when other features of collapse are present; a more subtle hilar abnormality (e.g. slight depression of the left hilum in early collapse of the left lower lobe resulting in both hilar shadows at the same level) may, however, be the only indication of early lobar collapse. The approximation of ribs as a feature of lobar collapse is of little diagnostic importance, its presence invariably being associated with the other features described above.

Further reading

CARLSON, V., MARTIN, J. E., KEEGAN, J. M. and DAILEY, J. E. (1966) Roentgenographic features of mucoid impaction of the bronchi. *American Journal of Roentgenology, Radium Therapy and Nuclear Medicine*, **96**, 947

SIMON, G. (1984) *Principles of Chest X-ray Diagnosis*. London: Butterworths

Answers—Plate 2

2.1 Thymoma.

2.2 Myasthenia gravis.

The postero-anterior radiograph (Plate 2a) shows a well-demarcated bi-lobed homogeneous shadow containing flecks of calcification. The lateral view (Plate 2b) shows a hazy opacity lying retrosternally, localizing the abnormality to the anterior mediastinum (see below). In the presence of symptoms suggesting myasthenia gravis, there is usually little doubt as to the nature of such a radiographic abnormality. About 15% of patients with this condition have thymomas, the onset of myasthenia usually, but not always, preceding the detection of the thymic tumour. Between 25% and 50% of all patients with thymic tumours have myasthenia and among myasthenic patients with a thymic tumour about half will show symptomatic improvement following thymectomy. The best results are achieved in younger patients and those with a short history of symptoms. Other causes of thymic enlargement include chronic haemolytic states, systemic lupus erythematosus, polymyositis and thyrotoxicosis.

Solid thymomas are the most frequently occurring anterior mediastinal neoplasms and are as often benign as malignant. They may occur at any age, but are rare in children. They are usually found near the junction of the heart and great vessels which are displaced posteriorly. They are typically smooth, well-demarcated and rounded or oval in shape, but may also be lobulated. They project to one or both sides of the mediastinum. Their size varies (usually 1–5 cm diameter) and they may be difficult to detect by conventional radiographic means. In these circumstances, computed tomography (CT) will often provide useful diagnostic information (Mink et al., 1978). Small central areas of calcification are typical but extensive and irregular 'woolly' calcification is also seen, and in some patients the thymic abnormality is cystic and shows peripheral curvilinear calcification. Although usually asymptomatic, thymomas may present with stridor, dyspnoea or sternal pain due to local pressure effects. A rapid increase in size and the presence of symptoms is suggestive of malignancy. Metastases are rare, but recurrence following surgical removal is not uncommon.

In all cases of mediastinal abnormality the lateral view radiograph plays an important role in differential diagnosis as it permits localization of the lesion. The mediastinum may be arbitrarily divided into four compartments: the superior compartment extending from the thoracic inlet above to a horizontal line drawn from the fifth thoracic vertebra to the manubrio-sternal joint below; the anterior compartment lying

Table 2* Causes of anterior mediastinal shadows

Relative position of shadow	Cause
Lying in a high position	Retrosternal thyroid
	Aneurysmal or tortuous innominate artery
	Post operative haematoma, e.g. thymectomy, cardiac surgery
Lying in upper three-quarters of anterior mediastinum	Lymphoproliferative disorders
	Non-malignant mediastinal lymphadenopathy
	Mediastinal abscess
	Dermoid cyst/teratoma
	Cystic hygroma
	Thymic cyst/tumour
	Secondary tumour deposits
	Ectopic thyroid
	Ectopic parathyroid
	Lipoma/other rare benign tumour
Lying in a low position, touching diaphragm	Pleural/pericardial cyst
	Morgagni hernia
	Pericardial fat pad

* Modified from Simon (1984)

68

anterior to the heart; the posterior compartment extending from the posterior aspect of the heart to the vertebrae and ribs; and the middle compartment occupied principally by the heart, great vessels and major bronchi. Certain lesions have a predilection for particular mediastinal compartments thus permitting a short list of diagnostic possibilities on anatomical grounds. The other radiographic features and the clinical context will usually allow precise diagnosis. Simon (1984) has subdivided the causes of anterior mediastinal shadows according to their relative location (Table 2). The detailed structure of many of these lesions is particularly well demonstrated by computed tomography which can play a useful role in differential diagnosis (*see* later).

References

MINK, J. H., BEIN, M. E., SUKOV, R. et al. (1978) Computed tomography of the anterior mediastinum in patients with myasthenia gravis and suspected thymoma. *American Journal of Roentgenology,* **130,** 239

SIMON, G. (1984) *Principles of Chest X-ray Diagnosis.* London: Butterworths

Answers—Plate 3

3.1 Right pneumothorax.
Bilateral diffuse reticular shadowing producing a honeycomb pattern.

3.2 Histiocytosis-X (eosinophilic granuloma)

The term 'honeycomb shadowing' is used to describe the radiographic appearance produced by closely set small ring shadows, each possessing a wall about 1–2 mm wide surrounding a circular central area of transradiancy 3–8 mm in diameter (Plate 3b). The term 'cystic lung' (coarse 'honeycomb shadowing') is sometimes used when the ring shadows are of large diameter (>1 cm).
Honeycomb shadowing can be the result of a range of lung pathology including cryptogenic fibrosing alveolitis, rheumatoid arthritis, systemic sclerosis, sarcoidosis, cystic fibrosis, pneumoconiosis and bronchiectasis. Extensive and uniform 'honeycombing' is, however, particularly suggestive of four disparate disease states: *Histiocytosis-X, Tuberous sclerosis, Lymphangiomyomatosis* and *Neurofibromatosis.* The clinical diagnosis of histiocytosis-X is suggested here by the presence

69

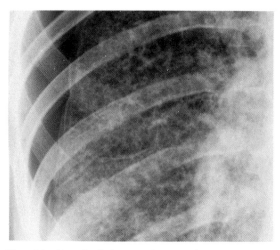

Plate 3*b*   Detail of plate 3*a* showing 'honeycombing' due to groups of closely set hairline ring shadows.

of thirst and polyuria due to co-existing diabetes insipidus, a characteristic associated abnormality. Sarcoidosis can also cause a destructive pituitary lesion but this is an unlikely cause of such a uniform pattern of 'honeycomb shadowing'. Lytic bone lesions, a feature in about 5–10% of patients with histiocytosis-X, are a useful diagnostic clue and the ribs, clavicles, scapulae, etc., should be carefully scrutinized for this reason.

The course of the disease is variable. In the case illustrated, there was relentless disease progression with increasing exertional dyspnoea. Prominence of the main pulmonary artery (Plate 3*a*) indicates a degree of pulmonary hypertension, a common accompaniment of advanced disease, which in this patient culminated in death from cor pulmonale. In the early stages of the disease the chest radiograph usually shows diffuse nodular shadowing corresponding to a pleomorphic cellular infiltrate in which abnormal histiocytes predominate and in which eosinophils are often prominent (hence the alternative descriptive term, eosinophilic granuloma). With progressive disease, disruption of alveolar septa and the development of cysts leads to the more characteristic radiographic appearance illustrated here. These dilated air spaces are especially liable to rupture and spontaneous

70

pneumothorax complicates the course of the disease in 20–30% of patients. Although particularly common in histiocytosis-X, the occurrence of pneumothorax has been described in many insterstitial disorders, generally in the later stages of the disease when extensive architectural distortion leads to rupture of subpleural cysts.

Further reading

LEWIS, J. G. (1964) Eosinophilic granuloma and its variants with special reference to lung involvement. *Quarterly Journal of Medicine*, **33**, 337

MASSARO, D., KATZ, S., MATTHEWS, M. J. and HIGGINS, G. (1975) Von Recklinghausens' neurofibromatosis associated with cystic lung disease. *American Journal of Medicine*, **38**, 233

STOVIN, P. G. I., LUM, L. C., FLOWER, C. D. R., DARKE, C. S. and BEELEY, M. (1975) The lungs in lymphangiomyomatosis and in tuberous sclerosis. *Thorax*, **30**, 497

Answers—Plate 4

4.1 Right upper-zone pulmonary hamartoma.

Hamartomas are tumours in which normal components of the organ are combined in a disorganized manner. Although considered to be congenital in origin, pulmonary hamartomas are rarely encountered in childhood and generally present in adult life, most commonly in the fourth decade. Two types are recognized: cartilaginous and fibroleiomyomatous.

Typically 2–3 cms in diameter, hamartomas vary greatly in size and may occupy the entire hemithorax (Petheram and Heard, 1979). They normally occur singly, but multiple pulmonary hamartomas are also described (Nili et al., 1979). Radiologically they usually show a circular or slightly lobulated outline with a well defined edge. Calcification occurs in a minority and may be difficult to detect on plain radiographs. When present calcification is characteristically central and frequently of the 'popcorn' variety, a feature best appreciated in tomograms (Plate 4b). A cystic appearance is sometimes noted owing to tumour necrosis or deposits of fat.

The vast majority of cases are diagnosed fortuitously in asymptomatic patients from routine chest radiographs which usually show a peripheral opacity. Some 3–5% of cartilaginous hamartomas and 50% of the fibroleiomyomatous variety occur intrabronchially and may present with haemoptysis or with symptoms or signs related to pulmonary infection or

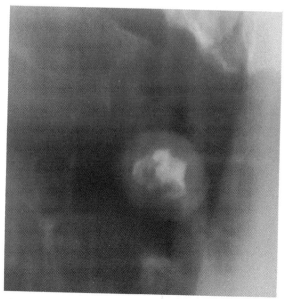

Plate 6b Pulmonary hamartoma: tomogram demonstrating characteristic central 'popcorn' calcification.

collapse. The latter type occurs in a diffuse form which may be associated with tuberous sclerosis and is one cause of 'honeycomb lung'. Malignant change may occur, but is rare and said not to occur in fibroleiomyomatous hamartomas.

A definite diagnosis is difficult to establish with certainty prior to thoracotomy although percutaneous needle biopsy may be helpful. Unless contraindicated by virtue of poor respiratory reserve, co-existing disease, etc., surgical resection is desirable, not least because of the difficulties in distinguishing non-calcified hamartomas from peripheral bronchial carcinomas. The tumours can often be 'shelled out' without sacrificing normal lung tissue. The postoperative prognosis is excellent.

References

NILI, M., VIDNE, B. A., AVIDOR, I., PAZ, R. and LEVY, M. (1979) Multiple pulmonary hamartomas; a case report and review of the literature. *Scandinavian Journal of Thoracic and Cardiovascular Surgery,* **13,** 157

PETHERAM, I. S. and HEARD, B. A. (1979) Unique massive pulmonary hamartoma. Case report with review of hamartomata treated at Brompton Hospital in 27 years. *Chest,* **75,** 95

Answers—Plate 5

5.1 Bilateral diffuse micronodular shadowing.
Bilateral well-defined areas of homogeneous shadowing occupying both upper zones.

5.2 Coalworkers' pneumoconiosis.
Progressive massive fibrosis.

'Simple' coalworkers' pneumoconiosis (CWP) is characterized radiographically by the presence of multiple small pulmonary opacities which are distributed diffusely throughout both lung fields. The opacities vary in size, being either punctiform (diameter up to 1.5 mm), micronodular (diameter 1.5–3 mm) or nodular (diameter 3–10 mm). Rounded micronodular opacities are usual in CWP. Irregular opacities are sometimes seen but are more common in pneumoconioses due to other causes, e.g. asbestosis. Simple CWP is probably not a cause of respiratory symptoms or disability. Its severity is determined purely on radiological grounds according to the profusion of opacities; the greater their profusion the greater the risk of progressive massive fibrosis. In general, the radiographic appearances do not change after cessation of exposure although, rarely, simple CWP may progress to progressive massive fibrosis (PMF) after exposure has ceased.

PMF (the development of progressive massive areas of fibrous tissue in the presence of pneumoconiosis) is most commonly recognized in association with CWP, although it can also complicate the course of silicosis and pneumoconioses due to haematite, kaolin and graphite. Early PMF causes no symptoms and little abnormality of lung function. More advanced PMF is associated initially with restriction of lung volumes, followed by progressive airways obstruction secondary to distortion of pulmonary architecture and recurrent infection. Progressive disability is the rule even after cessation of exposure.

Radiologically, PMF is recognized by the presence of rounded or oval homogeneous opacities (diameter >1 cm), usually bilateral and most often affecting the upper lobes. The lesions tend to be irregular and ill-defined in the early stages, but increase slowly in size over a period of years, become better defined and tend to migrate towards the hilum leaving an area of emphysematous lung peripherally.

The mass lesions of PMF require differentiation from bronchial carcinoma and tuberculosis. The shape of the masses is often helpful in this respect in that they tend to have a smooth lateral border, parallel to the rib cage and 1–3 cms from it on the postero-anterior film. The medial margin tends to be less well defined. These characteristics occurring against a background of simple pneumoconiosis and a history of occupational exposure will be strongly suggestive. The lesions may cavitate with the expectoration of jet black material (melanoptysis), pathognomonic for coalworkers' pneumoconiosis and therefore diagnostic in the present illustration.

Answers—Plate 6

6.1 Bilateral rib notching.
Coarctation of the aorta.

6.2 Hypertension; left ventricular failure; subacute bacterial endocarditis; cerebral haemorrhage from an associated 'berry' aneurysm; aortic rupture.

The rib notching (pressure erosion of the ribs) seen here is typical of that resulting from aortic coarctation, being bilateral, more or less symmetrical and most evident on the inferior aspect of the posterior parts of ribs 4–8. The first and second ribs are spared as their arteries are supplied by a branch of the subclavian. Plate 6b shows part of the left lung field in greater detail, illustrating the smooth, localized and curvilinear appearance of the erosions. These result from increased ('reversed') blood flow through dilated, tortuous intercostal arteries which take part in a collateral circulation between the subclavian artery and the aorta distal to the coarctation. Unilateral (right-sided) rib notching occurs when the coarctation is proximal to or at the level of the origin of the left subclavian artery. Unilateral (left-sided) rib notching is seen when an aberrant right subclavian artery, apparent on barium swallow, arises from the aorta distal to the coarctation. Rib notching is rarely present before the age of 10–12.

Other causes of rib notching include multiple intercostal neurofibromata (usually in association with generalized neurofibromatosis) and other conditions in which enlargement of intercostal nerves is a feature, e.g. amyloidosis, congenital hypertrophic polyneuropathy. A collateral circulation involving grossly dilated intercostal veins is a rare cause

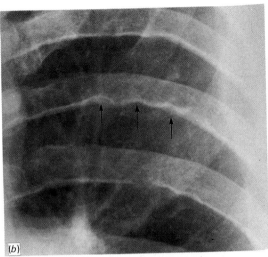

Plate 6b   Detail of the left lung field from Plate 6a showing smooth, localized, curvilinear rib erosions (arrowed) in aortic coarctation.

of rib notching, but has been described secondary to superior vena caval obstruction and in some cases of portal hypertension due to hepatic cirrhosis when oesophageal venous flow is greatly increased. Unilateral rib notching is also seen after a Blalock anastomosis for Fallot's tetralogy: following anastomosis of the left subclavian and left main pulmonary arteries, diminished blood flow to the left arm encourages a collateral circulation via the intercostal arteries supplying the distal left subclavian artery. Rib notching is occasionally congenital in origin. Other rare causes include arterio-venous fistulae, pulmonary oligaemia (e.g. due to pulmonary atresia) and obstructive arteritis (e.g. Takayasu's disease).

A variety of radiographic abnormalities other than rib notching may be seen (Table 3). Among these, variations in the size and shape of the aortic knuckle are the most constant. Most commonly the aortic knuckle is elongated, higher than normal and runs into the shadow of the dilated left subclavian artery. A penetrated radiograph may be required to visualize the post-stenotic dilatation of the descending aorta which displaces the barium filled oesophagus to the right. Left ventricular hypertrophy occurs due to pressure overload, but cardiac enlargement is often not apparent or, if present, only

Table 3 Radiographic abnormalities in coarctation of the aorta

Rib notching
Small aortic knuckle
Various abnormalities of the shape of the aortic knuckle, e.g. flattened lateral
    aspect or shallow lateral concave notch
Dilated left subclavian artery producing a left paravertebral shadow in the left
    superior mediastinum
Post-stenotic dilatation of the descending aorta
Prominent ascending aorta
Cardiomegaly

slight unless aortic valve disease co-exists or heart failure supervenes.

About 60% of all adults with coarctation are asymptomatic and the diagnosis is established at a routine medical examination. About 10% of patients have an associated aortic valve lesion. Other associations include ventricular septal defect and Turner's syndrome. Systolic hypertension limited to the upper extremities is characteristic of adult coarctation. About one quarter of all patients die from hypertensive complications (cardiac failure, cerebral haemorrhage). Subacute bacterial endocarditis is less common than previously as a cause of death. The usual site of infection is the aortic valve which is often bicuspid. A similar clinical picture is produced by bacterial aortitis arising in the aortic intima just distal to the coarctation or occasionally in the ascending aorta. Aortic rupture, the cause of death in about 25% of cases, may occur just above the aortic valve or just below the site of the coarctation where post-stenotic dilatation can reach aneurysmal proportions.

Answers—Plate 7

7.1 Dermoid cyst.

7.2 Infection.
Malignant change.

There is a well circumscribed homogeneous opacity of soft tissue density situated medially in the right middle and lower zones, overlying the right heart border. Centrally, there are scattered flecks of calcification and, peripherally, there is a rim of curvilinear calcification. The lateral view radiograph shows the mass lying anteriorly in the mediastinum (see Table 2, p.68), superimposed upon the cardiac shadow. These appearances in an asymptomatic patient strongly suggest a dermoid cyst as the most likely cause of the opacity. The nature of the lesion is obvious when bone or teeth are present, elements which may be seen in the plain radiograph but which are most clearly demonstrated by tomography, particularly computed tomography, the value of which in the differential diagnosis of mediastinal masses has already been referred to (see Question 2).

The dermoid is a tumour of developmental origin in which normal components of the organ and components not normally represented in the lung are combined in a disorganized manner. Dermoids vary in size (up to 12 cm diameter) and configuration. Typically cystic rather than solid and rounded or ovoid in outline, they are occasionally lobulated and multilocular. Their dense fibrous capsules are lined by stratified squamous epithelium. Although all three germinal layers are usually represented, tissues are largely of ectodermal origin. Typical contents include sebaceous material with elements of skin, hair, teeth, bone, cartilage, neural tissue, intestinal and bronchial epithelium and occasionally muscle, usually of the smooth variety. Some authors suggest that the term 'dermoid cyst' be reserved for cases where the mass consists only of epidermis and its appendages and that the term 'teratoma' be applied to cases where all three germinal layers are represented. Others use the term 'teratodermoid' to overcome this difficulty.

Dermoids are usually asymptomatic until complications occur. Occasionally symptoms arise from the large size of some lesions causing local compression of adjacent viscera and resulting in, for example, substernal pain, dyspnoea, cough or stridor and, rarely, with very large tumours, dysphagia from oesophageal compression. The expectoration of hair (trichoptysis) is pathognomonic but rare.

Symptoms are usually the result of either malignant change or infection. The former arises in about 30% of dermoids and occurs almost exclusively in males. Infection transforms the dermoid into an abscess which may rupture into the pleura or into a bronchus, the resulting fistula transforming the radiographic picture with the appearance of an air-fluid level. Surrounding inflammation imparts an irregular outline to the periphery of the normally well-demarcated lesion.

Answers—Plate 8

8.1 Ill-defined left mid-zone consolidation.
   Left hilar lymphadenopathy.
   Right paratracheal lymphadenopathy.

8.2 Primary pulmonary tuberculosis.

The patient was X-rayed as a contact of her father who had been diagnosed as having open pulmonary tuberculosis. About 3.5% of domestic contacts of an index case are found to have active tuberculosis, the likelihood of infection being greatest in contacts of smear positive patients. In adolescents and young adults, whereas some primary infections present with malaise or respiratory symptoms secondary to bronchial involvement (relating to the lymph node component of the disease), the majority of cases are asymptomatic. Untreated, most cases will resolve without complications and the primary focus heals completely. In a proportion of cases the lesion progresses when infection may spread via the bronchi leading to tuberculous bronchopneumonia, via the lymphatics to the pleura resulting in a pleural effusion, or via the bloodstream with miliary spread or other haematogeneous forms of tuberculosis (renal, joint, bone, etc.) as possible consequences. The risk of dissemination, especially in younger age groups, or of progressive pulmonary disease in older individuals is sufficient, therefore, to justify antituberculous chemotherapy in all cases where there is a radiographically visible lesion.

The two components of the primary complex, pulmonary and glandular, produce variable radiographic appearances. In adults the pulmonary abnormality is usually obvious and is most often situated in the upper zone. When it is less clearly seen, tomography permits more accurate evaluation of the lung lesion. The glandular component is frequently inapparent leading to confusion with post-primary tuberculosis. Therefore, unless it is known that the patient has recently become tuberculin positive, the distinction between primary and post-primary tuberculosis may be difficult. In children the pulmonary component may occur in any part of the lung and varies greatly in extent, from being undetectable to causing extensive caseous pneumonia. Hilar lymphadenopahy tends to be more obvious than in adults and may be marked or associated with paratracheal lymph node enlargement.

Affected nodes in close relation to the superior vena cava constitute a special danger, being a likely precursor of miliary tuberculosis. Lymphadenopathy is also frequently pronounced in patients of Asian extraction belonging to any age group. Radiographic changes of collapse or consolidation may result when caseous nodes compress or discharge into a segmental or lobar bronchus. Partial bronchial obstruction may cause a valve action with trapping of air within a lung segment or lobe producing an area of localized hypertransradiancy ('obstructive' emphysema) on the chest radiograph, a rare complication occurring most commonly in children under two years of age.

Resolution of the primary infection is often accompanied by calcification affecting one or both components of the primary complex when the radiographic appearances are again often characteristic (Plate 8b). In the example shown, the glandular component of the infection had also involved cervical lymph nodes.

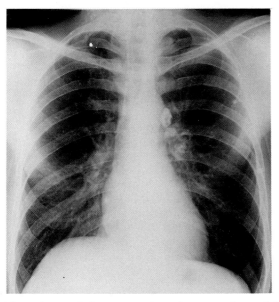

Plate 8b Healed primary tuberculous complex: calcified left hilar lymph nodes. Small, peripheral left mid-zone calcific density. Note also scattered right-sided cervical calcification.

Answers—Plate 9

9.1 Wegener's granulomatosis.

Wegener's granulmatosis forms part of a spectrum of diseases the characteristic feature of which is a necrotizing vasculitis. It is distinguished from other forms of 'polyarteritis' by the involvement of small vessels, including both arteries and veins. Lesions predominate in the upper and lower respiratory tract, which together with a focal necrotizing glomerulonephritis are the classical clinical manifestations. 'Classical' polyarteritis nodosa affects medium-sized arteries and pulmonary involvement is comparatively rare.

Almost all patients with pulmonary involvement also have disease affecting the upper airways. Typically, patients present with nasal symptoms of prolonged duration, but the middle ear, paranasal sinuses and larynx may all be involved. Nasal discharge, occasionally colourless at first, is usually purulent and may be bloodstained. Ultimately, the destructive granulomatous process, which may extend into the orbits, frequently results in a typical saddle nose deformity.

Pulmonary involvement produces a wide range of clinical and radiographic manifestations. Granulomatous lesions may involve bronchial walls resulting in radiographic evidence of segmental or lobar collapse. More commonly, intrapulmonary lesions give rise to multiple, rounded, homogeneous densities, 1–10 cm in diameter (see Plate 9), showing a marked tendency to cavitate. The lesions are often transient and may resolve in one area only to be replaced by similar lesions in another part of the lung. They are usually well defined and there may be some difficulty in distinguishing them from pulmonary metastases. Other radiographic features include areas of segmental consolidation due to pulmonary infarction, occasional small pleural effusions and, less commonly, evidence of secondary infection.

Any system may be involved in classical Wegener's granulomatosis, but the prognosis is most closely related to the presence and severity of associated renal involvement. In the absence of treatment, mean survival after the appearance of clinical evidence of renal disease is only five months. Immunosuppressive therapy will induce long-term remissions in most patients and will cure some. Cyclophosphamide is the drug of choice. Corticosteroids are usually given, but are possibly best reserved for when there is evidence of ocular or (severe) serosal involvement and then given in short courses along with cyclophosphamide.

Further reading

FAUCI, A. S. and WOLFF, S. M. (1973) Wegener's granulomatosis: Studies in eighteen patients and a review of the literature. *Medicine*, **52**, 535

Answers—Plate 10

10.1 Allergic bronchopulmonary aspergillosis.

10.2 Skin prick test to *Aspergillus fumigatus* (*Asp. fumigatus*) antigen.
Peripheral blood eosinophil count.
Determination of serum precipitating antibody to *Asp. fumigatus*.
Sputum culture for *Aspergillus* species.

The first film (Plate 10a) shows bilateral perihilar shadowing most marked on the right and a group of band-like shadows in the right lower zone adjacent to the cardiac border. Ten days later (Plate 10b) the radiographic appearances have changed dramatically. Left-sided perihilar consolidation is now more prominent, whilst that on the right has shown marked resolution. In addition, the lower-zone, band-like shadows have been replaced by parallel-line shadows with a central transradiant zone (*see* below). These radiographic abnormalities in an asthmatic patient are characteristic of pulmonary eosinophilia which in 'extrinsic' asthma is most commonly the result of allergic bronchopulmonary aspergillosis (ABPA).

The transient radiographic shadows of ABPA are of two main types. The first group results from pulmonary eosinophilic 'pneumonia' and, typically, these shadows consist of non-segmental areas of homogeneous consolidation, frequently perihilar in distribution, affecting the upper lobes predominantly and often extremely transient, sometimes resolving after only one or two days. The second group of shadows represents manifestations of bronchial obstruction or dilatation and consists of various types of 'tubular' shadow. Band-like shadows as in Plate 10a are seen when secretions

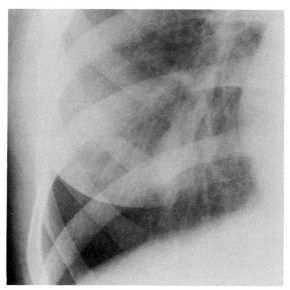

Plate 10c   Allergic bronchopulmonary aspergillosis: 'gloved finger' shadow.

fill a dilated bronchus; these may be referred to as 'toothpaste' shadows when the walls are truly parallel, or 'gloved finger' shadows when there is distal globular enlargement (Plate 10c). Despite the presence of segmental bronchial occlusion by fluid or mucus, collapse is not a feature owing to the existence of communications – the Pores of Kohn and the Canals of Lambert – between the affected lung and the alveoli or bronchioli of adjacent lung segments. This phenomenon ('collateral air drift') does not prevent lobar collapse because the pulmonary lobes are bounded by the visceral pleura. Parallel line shadows are the result of peribronchial thickening affecting dilated but patent bronchi. Their appearance characteristically follows the expectoration of purulent sputum plugs, which are a feature in about one third of patients with ABPA and which may be responsible for recurrent episodes of lobar or even pulmonary collapse (Ellis, 1965).

   Repeated episodes of pulmonary eosinophilia and the tissue damaging reactions, mediated by precipitating antibody (Arthus type III reactions), with which they are associated,

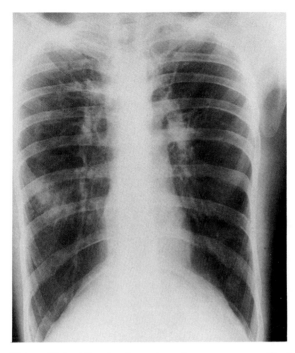

Plate 10*d* Allergic bronchopulmonary aspergillosis: aerated shrunken upper lobes with upward hilar retraction; note also the area of consolidation in right middle and lower zones.

lead to permanent radiographic abnormalities. Aerated but shrunken upper lobes may be seen (plate 10*d*), similar to the appearances in the extrinsic allergic alveolitis of bird fancier's lung. In some patients recurrent damage to bronchial walls leads to a characteristic form of saccular bronchiectasis (Plate 10*e*) involving proximal bronchi which show normal distal filling at bronchography. This contrasts with the more usual bronchographic appearance of bronchiectasis complicating tuberculosis or pyogenic infection, where contrast fails to fill the distal segments of affected bronchi.

The major criteria required for the diagnosis of ABPA are: a history of asthma; recurrent radiographic shadowing; peripheral blood eosinophilia (usually modest, e.g. 0.6–1.5 $\times$ 10^9/l); and a positive immediate skin prick test to *Asp. fumigatus* antigen. It is characteristic of the condition,

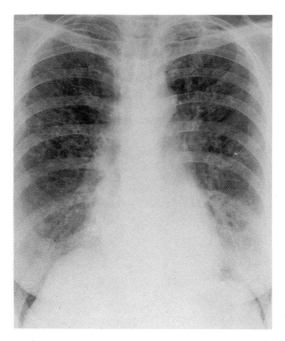

Plate 10e Allergic bronchopulmonary aspergillosis – saccular bronchiectasis: well defined ring shadows (most evident in right mid-zone) due to dilatation of proximal bronchi.

however, that the diagnostic features are variable and intermittent. Asthmatic symptoms are not prominent in all patients and the episodes of pulmonary eosinophilia are not always closely related to exacerbations of asthma. The mere present of *Aspergillus* species in the sputum does not replace evidence of allergy as a major criterion. *Asp. fumugatus* will often colonize the bronchial tree as a non-specific feature in a variety of chronic bronchopulmonary disorders. Further, in ABPA, the fungus may be seen or grown from sputum only intermittently. The presence of serum precipitins correlates well with a delayed positive (Arthus type) skin test reaction with *Asp. fumigatus* antigen, but their demonstration is also variable and closely dependent upon laboratory technique.

References

ELLIS, R. H. (1965) Total collapse of the lung in aspergillosis. *Thorax*, **20**, 118

Further reading

McCARTHY, D. S. and PEPYS, J. (1971) Allergic Bronchopulmonary aspergillosis. Clinical Immunology: (1) Clinical features. *Clinical Allergy,* **1,** 261

McCARTHY, D. S., SIMON, G. and HARGREAVE, F. E. (1970) The radiological appearances in allergic broncho-pulmonary aspergillosis. *Clinical Radiology,* **21,** 366

Answers—Plate 11

11.1 Left ventricular aneurysm.

11.2 In this patient syncopal episodes were related to recurrent ventricular tachycardia. Angina pectoris, cardiac failure, systemic embolism and, occasionally, pericarditis with or without an effusion may also be presenting features. Cardiac rupture is a rare occurrence.

There is a localized hump altering the normally smooth regular outline of the left heart border. Such an appearance is seen in about 50% of cases of left ventricular aneurysm. There is usually cardiomegaly but a normal cardiac size and outline in the postero-anterior film does not exclude the diagnosis. As it increases in size the aneurysm characteristically extends laterally and superiorly and in Plate 11a an obvious abnormality is present. Plate 11b shows the radiographic appearance in the same patient 12 months earlier when there is no prominent bulge, but a sharp angulation transforming the cardiac contour into a more oblong shape which may be likened to the toe of a well-worn boot. The location of the aneurysm in this example (i.e. where the more horizontal part of the left heart border turns downwards) is typical of most. They are often best seen in oblique projections and may be particularly well demarcated following the deposition of calcium in their walls. Paradoxical pulsation is often evident on fluoroscopy, but more precise delineation of the extent of the aneurysm requires echocardiography, radionuclide ventriculography or cine-angiocardiography, during which the affected segment of the left ventricle appears either akinetic (no movement during systole) or dyskinetic (abnormal, sometimes paradoxical, movement during systole).

The majority of cardiac aneurysms result from myocardial infarction. Rarely, they have an infective (e.g. syphilitic, mycotic or complicating bacterial endocarditis), congenital or

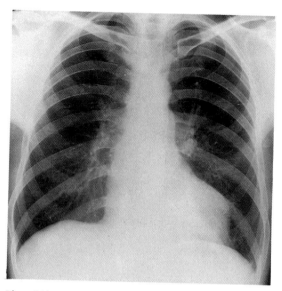

Plate 11*b* Postero-anterior film taken 12 months before that shown in Plate 11*a*. Note the 'sawn-off' appearance of the left ventricular outline.

traumatic aetiology. Most are small. Clinically significant aneurysms are uncommon.

The presence of the aneurysm does not in itself materially influence the prognosis of the original myocardial infarction. Angina pectoris is usually simply a reflection of underlying coronary artery disease and is seldom directly attributable to the aneurysm *per se*. Aneurysmal rupture virtually never occurs, while systemic embolism is probably no more frequent than after myocardial infarction without aneurysm formation. Surgery is indicated for large aneurysms causing left ventricular failure and when systemic embolism is not prevented by adequate anticoagulant therapy. Rarely, surgery may also be necessary for uncontrollable ventricular dysrhythmias.

Further reading

GOLDBERG, M. J. (1982) Left ventricular aneurysm. *British Journal of Hospital Medicine*, **27,** 143

Answers—Plate 12

12.1 Left upper lobe collapse.

12.2 A benign intrabronchial tumour.

The hazy appearance of the left hemithorax is characteristic and results from the superimposition of the collapsed upper lobe upon the overinflated portion of the apical segment of the left lower lobe. Loss of volume is reflected in slight elevation of the left dome of the diaphragm and upward displacement of the left hilum, the outline of which is also abnormal – the lateral convexity being due to the rotated position of the basal artery. The lower margin of the homogeneous opacity is poorly defined, whilst the left heart border is also indistinct owing to lingular involvement, an example of the 'silhouette sign'. The loss of a normally visible silhouette in the anterior view radiograph indicates that two structures of the same radiographic density lie in the same plane. The left heart border is normally clearly defined because it lies adjacent to the expanded lingular segment of the left upper lobe, which is of 'air density'. When the lingula is consolidated or collapsed it acquires the same ('soft tissue') radiographic density as the heart, the silhouette of which is then lost. In some cases of upper lobe collapse the lingular segment is spared and the left ventricular outline remains well defined (Plate 12b).

The characteristics of left upper lobe collapse contrast sharply with those of collapse involving the right upper lobe owing to the absence of a minor fissure in the left lung. The radiological diagnosis is readily confirmed by the lateral view radiograph (Plate 12c). The lobe collapses in an anterior and superomedial direction and is bounded posteriorly by the displaced oblique fissure (arrowed). Anteriorly, the tongue-like shadow of the collapsed lobe either reaches the sternum or, as in Plate 12c, lies slightly posteriorly to it when the intervening transradiant area is occupied by that part of the right lung which has herniated across the midline.

Benign tumours of the respiratory tract are uncommon, having an incidence somewhat less than 1% of primary bronchial carcinomas. They encompass a wide range of histology: adenomas, leiomyomas, lipomas, fibromas, chondromas, chemodectomas, etc. Of those tumour types arising within the bronchial tree, bronchial adenomas are the most

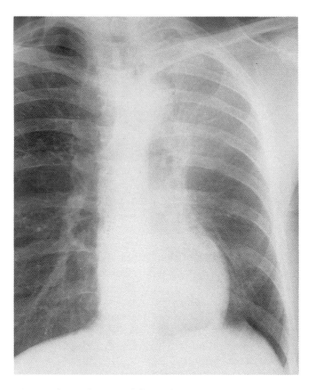

Plate 12*b* Left upper lobe collapse sparing the lingula: left heart border remains well defined.

common. Two histological varieties are recognized – 'carcinoid' tumours (80–90% of adenomas) and 'cylindromas'. Although described as benign, adenomas have the potential for malignant transformation (greater in the case of 'cylindromas'), which is sometimes evident after several years of non-invasive growth.

Bronchial adenomas show an equal sex incidence and a peak age incidence in the second or third decade. The majority of adenomas (~75%) arise centrally, within large airways, and the leading symptoms are haemoptysis and symptoms related to bronchial obstruction. The slow intra-bronchial growth of the tumour not infrequently results in repeated episodes of pneumonia affecting the same pulmonary segment or lobe over a period of months or years – a

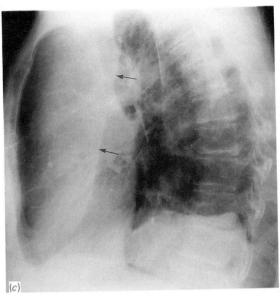

Plate 12c Left upper lobe collapse – lateral view radiograph: posterior border of collapsed lobe demarcated by displaced oblique fissure (arrowed).

presentation which, especially in a young non-smoker, should suggest the diagnosis. Surgery is indicated even in the absence of infective complications because of the potential risk of malignant change. The fundamentally benign nature of the tumour dictates a far less radical approach than that required in bronchial carcinoma.

Further reading

MARKS, C. and MARKS, M. (1977) Bronchial adenoma. A clinicopathological study. *Chest*, **71,** 376

Answers—Plate 13

13.1 Pleuropericardial cyst.

Pleuropericardial cysts represent congenital malformations arising during embryological development of the mediastinum. They are relatively uncommon with an estimated

89

incidence of 1 per 100 000 of the population, but must be considered in the differential diagnosis of anterior mediastinal masses (Table 2; p.68). Radiographically, the appearance is often characteristic: a smooth, rounded homogeneous density containing no calcification and located (in the anterior view) in the cardiophrenic angle. The lateral view radiograph confirms the anterior position of the mass, which is situated in the angle between the diaphragm and the sternum. About 70% are right-sided and therefore plainly visible on the postero-anterior film, whereas left-sided lesions are obscured by the cardiac shadow. Typically 2–3 cm in diameter, they may be as large as 10 cm.

Epicardial fat pads which are far commoner than pericardial cysts cause a very similar radiographic appearance as does a hernia through the foramen of Morgagni. In this latter case the distinction is possible when the Morgagni hernia contains a loop of bowel, producing an air transradiancy within the opacity. Alternatively, barium studies may be necessary for differentiation. When the hernia contains liver, hepatic ultrasound examination or an isotope liver scan will often prove diagnostic. Fat pads, Morgagni herniae and pleuroperi-cardial cysts are most readily differentiated, however, by

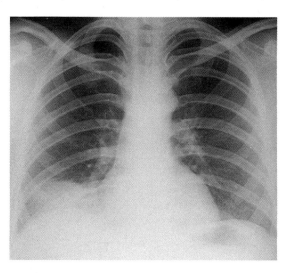

Plate 13c Pleuropericardial cyst: well-defined right lower zone opacity occupying cardiophrenic angle.

computed tomography (CT) which gives a measurement of the attenuation coefficient of an area of interest selected from the scan and, therefore, provides a rough estimate of the density of a lesion. Water has been arbitrarily assigned a CT number (tissue density) of 0. Relative to this and using Hounsfield units, air has a CT number of -1000, bone from $+200$ to $+2000$, fat -80 to -100 and other soft tissues $+10$ to $+80$. Lipomas, fat pads and dermoid cysts have a negative CT number. Soft tissue abnormalities and most fluid containing cysts (some are 'water dense', i.e. CT number 0) have a positive CT number. The CT value of vascular lesions characteristically increases following the intravenous injection of contrast medium, whereas that of fluid containing cysts does not change. This application of CT is illustrated by Plates 13c and 13d. The postero-anterior chest radiograph shows a well defined shadow occupying the right cardiophrenic angle. The corresponding CT scan shows a multiloculated lesion lying anteriorly adjacent to the right heart border. The CT number was $+3$ indicating a fluid containing pericardial cyst.

Histologically pleuropericardial cysts are benign structures having a thin, fibrous, outer wall and an inner lining composed of flattened mesothelial cells. Their characteristic content of clear colourless fluid is responsible for the

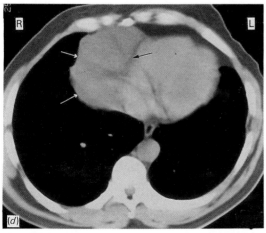

Plate 13d   Pleuropericardial cyst: thoracic CT scan corresponding to chest film in Plate 13c showing well demarcated, multilocular opacity (arrows) of water density (CT number $+3$).

alternative description, 'springwater cysts'. Malignant change does not occur and infection is a very rare complication. Almost invariably, therefore, they are symptomless and their benign nature is confirmed when comparison with a previous chest film (if available), taken some time before, shows no change in the appearances. When the diagnosis is beyond reasonable doubt surgical treatment is unnecessary unless infection supervenes.

Answers—Plate 14

14.1 Bilateral apical pleural thickening; left apical cavity containing a solid mass (mycetoma); upward retraction of the left hilum; linear shadowing and scattered calcification in the right middle and upper zones.

14.2 Sputum examination for tubercle bacilli and *Aspergillus* species; serum *Aspergillus* precipitins; sputum cytology for malignant cells; bronchoscopy.

In this patient haemoptysis was secondary to the left apical mycetoma. Investigations including bronchoscopy revealed no evidence of bronchial carcinoma or active tuberculosis, both clearly important considerations in a middle-aged smoker with radiographic evidence of previous tuberculous infection. The mycetoma shows the classical radiographic features: a well-defined ring shadow with a central homogeneous opacity representing the fungus ball; the latter does not completely fill the cavity and is separated from its wall by a transradiant zone of air – the so called 'halo shadow'. The typical features are best demonstrated by tomography (Plate 14*b*). Characteristically, the position of the fungus ball varies with the posture of the patient. Because it occupies the most dependent part of the cavity a superior crescentic air transradiancy (Plate 14*a*) is present when the patient is erect; with the patient supine as during antero-posterior tomography the transradiant zone of air is circular and completely surrounds the fungus ball. Rarely, an air space is not easily recognizable either on the plain radiograph or in tomograms.

Aspergillus fumigatus is by far the commonest fungus implicated in mycetoma formation. The vast majority occur in the apical segments of the upper lobes, a reflection of the fact

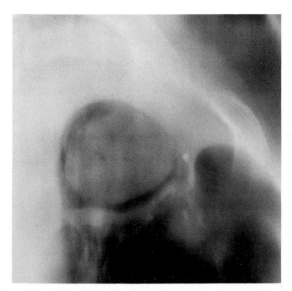

Plate 14b Mycetoma: antero-posterior tomogram showing thickened apical pleura and large cavity containing fungus ball surrounded by circular transradiant zone of air.

that most arise as a result of fungal colonization of healed tuberculous cavities. This was the most common (28% of cases) predisposing lung pathology in a recent series of 85 patients with pulmonary aspergilloma (Jewkes et al., 1983). Other causes of upper lobe fibrosis, sarcoidosis and allergic bronchopulmonary aspergillosis occurred commonly, but a wide variety of pre-existing pulmonary disorders including bullous emphysema, bronchiectasis, pneumonia and lung abscess may also predipose to the development of a mycetoma. In about 20% of cases aspergillomas are multiple. Serum precipitins to *Asp. fumigatus* are almost invariable. Immediate skin prick tests are positive in about 70% of cases. Asthmatic features are common and a small proportion of patients (ten out of 85 in Jewkes' series) satisfy the criteria for allergic bronchopulmonary aspergillosis.

Aspergillomas are frequently asymptomatic, but haemoptysis occurs at some stage in the majority of patients and may be life threatening in as many as 20% (Karas et al., 1976). In most patients cough and dyspnoea, which are common accompanying features, are related to the underlying lung disease. In a small proportion of patients, usually with large mycetomas, there is associated malaise, weight loss, febrile symptoms and occasionally marked cachexia. Invasive aspergillosis complicating aspergilloma is probably a rare occurrence, but its exact frequency is disputed.

The available treatments for aspergilloma are not satisfactory. Surgery has been recommended for recurrent haemoptysis, but is seldom feasible owing to the severity of co-existing pulmonary disease. Even among relatively fit patients surgery is associated with an operative mortality of about 7% and major complications (haemorrhage, bronchopleural fistula, empyema) in a similar proportion of patients. Intracavitary instillation of antifungal drugs has given variable results, while systemic antifungal therapy is without benefit except in the rare event of associated invasive aspergillosis (Rafferty et al., 1983). Recurrent severe haemoptysis in patients unfit for surgery can sometimes be successfully treated by bronchial arterial embolization.

In addition to mycetomas, pulmonary infection with *Aspergillus* species may cause three alternative types of clinical disorder: allergic bronchopulmonary aspergillosis, disseminated aspergillosis usually in immuno-compromised individuals and locally invasive *Aspergillus* infection associated with pulmonary necrosis.

References and further reading

JEWKES, J., KAY, P. H., PANETH, M. and CITRON, K. (1983) Pulmonary aspergilloma: analysis of prognosis in relation to haemoptysis and survey of treatment. *Thorax*, **38,** 572

RAFFERTY, P., BIGGS, B. A., CROMPTON, G. K. and GRANT, I. W. B. (1983). What happens to patients with pulmonary aspergilloma? Analysis of 23 cases. *Thorax*, **38,** 579

A REPORT FROM THE RESEARCH COMMITTEE OF THE BRITISH THORACIC AND TUBERCULOSIS ASSOCIATION. (1970). Aspergilloma and residual tuberculous cavities – the results of a resurvey. *Tubercle*, **51,** 227

Answers—Plate 15

15.1 Bilateral mammary implants

There are bilateral rounded homogeneous opacities in the middle and lower zones superimposed upon the breast shadows. The presence of normal lung vascular markings and the fact that the heart border is clearly defined (and therefore

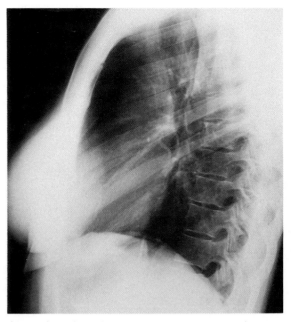

Plate 15b Bilateral mammary implants: lateral view radiograph –
areas of abnormal opacity are confined within margins of breast
shadows.

has aerated lung in contact with it) point away from an
intrapulmonary cause for the shadowing. The lateral view
radiograph (Plate 15b) clearly shows the areas of abnormal
opacity confined within the breast shadows. In general bizarre
appearances such as this, especially when symmetrical or
when associated with perfectly geometric outlines, should
suggest the possibility of artefact. Other common artefacts
include articles of clothing and plaits of hair in young women.
The latter may cast puzzling shadows over the upper zones of
the lungs, but their true nature can be determined if their
outline is traceable beyond the limits of the thorax.

The chest radiograph will occasionally show asymmetrical
breast shadows in patients with carcinoma of the breast (Plate
15c), while a previous mastectomy results in hypertransradiancy in the middle and lower zones relative to the opposite
normal hemithorax. Some normal breast shadows will also
occasionally produce diagnostic difficulty, as for example in

95

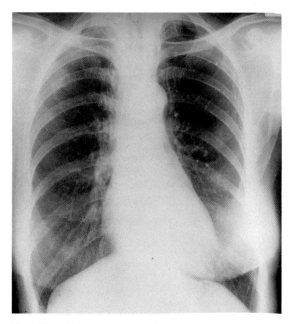

Plate 15c Postero-anterior chest radiograph showing asymmetrical breast shadows. Increased density in the left lower zone projects beyond the margin of the chest wall due to a carcinoma of the left breast.

thin, elderly women when rather fibrotic atrophic breast tissue may case somewhat unusual shadows (Plate 18b). The nature of the shadow is appreciated when it can be traced laterally to merge with the shadow of the lower axillary fold.

Answers—Plate 16

16.1 Pulmonary asbestosis.

16.2 Bilateral basal (late) inspiratory crackles on chest auscultation; finger clubbing.

There is ill-defined loss of translucency in both lower zones and close examination reveals a combination of irregular nodular opacities and short line shadows. In addition there is bilateral lower zone pleural thickening with blunting of the costophrenic angles. Calcification affecting the left hilar lymph nodes is an incidental abnormality due to healed primary tuberculosis.

The radiographic features of asbestosis are essentially similar to those of cryptogenic fibrosing alveolitis, i.e. bilateral reticulo-nodular shadowing with a lower zone predominance. The clinical signs (finger clubbing, basal lung crackles) are also identical, and in the absence of histological confirmation the diagnosis of asbestosis will often rest upon a history of occupational asbestos exposure. In contrast to cryptogenic fibrosing alveolitis, however, asbestosis is associated with pleural abnormalities in about 60% of cases. Thus, the presence of pleural thickening or pleural plaques provides indirect evidence that bilateral pulmonary fibrosis is causally related to asbestos.

The earliest radiographic evidence of asbestosis consists of small linear shadows of varying thickness (usually 1–3 mm) with lower zone predominance. In contrast the radiographic changes in silicosis show a characteristic middle and upper zone distribution. As with other forms of pneumoconiosis the radiographic extent of the disease is described according to an internationally agreed classification (International Labour Organization, 1980) by reference to a set of standard films. Characteristically, increasing profusion of the shadows obscures the intrapulmonary vascular pattern and the outlines of the heart and diaphragm become less distinct. With progression of pulmonary fibrosis, irregular nodular shadows increase in profusion and, occasionally, these predominate over linear shadows in the earlier stages of the disease. Ultimately, advanced pulmonary fibrosis with the formation of cysts, 'honeycombing' and the radiographic features of pulmonary hypertension supervene. Large confluent areas of fibrosis similar to those seen in coalworker's pneumoconiosis (see Question 5) may also complicate asbestosis, but this is relatively rare.

The severity of the disease and the proportion of affected workers varies with the intensity of dust exposure. The incidence of asbestosis has steadily declined and in recent years the number of new certified cases throughout Britain has averaged about 150 per year. Patients present with effort dyspnoea. Pulmonary function testing characteristically shows a restrictive ventilatory defect with reduced lung volumes and impaired gas transfer capacity. Progressive fibrosis which may continue after asbestos exposure has ceased results in increasing disability and death, in uncomplicated cases, from respiratory failure and cor pulmonale. More than half of all patients with pulmonary asbestosis die, however, from bronchial carcinoma (see Question 24).

Further reading

FLETCHER, D. E. and EDGE, J. R. (1970) The early radiological changes in pulmonary and pleural asbestosis. *Clinical Radiology,* **21,** 355

INTERNATIONAL LABOUR ORGANIZATION, (1980) *International Classification of Radiographs of the Pneumoconioses.* ILO: Geneva

SOUTAR, C. A., SIMON, G. and TURNER-WARWICK, M. (1974) The radiology of asbestos-induced disease of the lungs. *British Journal of Diseases of the Chest,* **68,** 235

Answers—Plate 17

17.1 Bilateral hilar and paratracheal lymphadenopathy.

17.2 Sarcoidosis; tuberculosis and some other bacterial infections, e.g. whooping cough; viral infections, e.g. infectious mononucleosis; fungal infections, e.g. histoplasmosis; silicosis; berylliosis; malignant lymphoma and leukaemia; metastatic neoplasms; drug idiosyncrasy.

The radiographic appearance of bilateral hilar lymphadenopathy (BHL) is distinctive when the enlarged nodes are set out from the hilar regions such that a rim of transradiant lung separates them from the mediastinum. Enlargement of both main pulmonary arteries produces a superficially similar appearance. Differentiation is often possible from the plain radiograph as enlarged nodes generally show well defined, convex lateral and inferior margins. Where doubt remains, glandular and vascular causes of hilar enlargement can be readily distinguished by tomography.

Plate 17 shows bilateral hilar enlargement and widening of the superior mediastinal shadow with a lobulated contour, the appearances being consistent with enlargement of the bronchopulmonary (hilar), paratracheal and tracheobronchial lymph nodes. In sarcoidosis (the cause of the changes in this illustration), hilar lymph node enlargement is roughly symmetrical. Associated paratracheal lymphadenopathy (usually right sided) is present in excess of 50% of cases. It is usually less obvious, but occasionally overshadows the hilar component and, rarely, may occur in the absence of hilar node enlargement. Lymph node enlargement tends to be moderate and is seldom massive. Unilateral involvement is unusual.

By contrast unilateral hilar lymphadenopathy is the rule in primary pulmonary tuberculosis (see Question 8), while the strongly positive tuberculin reaction is in contradistinction to the tuberculin anergy that characterizes sarcoidosis. Adenopathy in whooping cough pneumonia is usually also unilateral, while that in infectious mononucleosis is typically bilateral and chiefly affects the hilar nodes. Associated splenomegaly, also a feature of sarcoidosis, may be noticeable on the chest radiograph.

Silicosis may produce bilateral hilar lymphadenopathy and in rare instances this is found in the absence of pulmonary parenchymal shadowing. A distinctive form of 'eggshell' calcification is characteristic although, rarely, this is also a feature of sarcoidosis. Chronic beryllium disease produces identical clinical and radiological features to those described in sarcoidosis, but there is usually a clear history of relevant occupational exposure.

In malignant lymphomas lymphadenopathy is usually bilateral, but is often asymmetrical, the paratracheal and tracheobronchial nodes being involved more often than hilar nodes which are seldom involved in isolation. Mediastinal and hilar node involvement in leukaemia is usually symmetrical and is much commoner in lymphatic than myeloid leukaemia.

Rarely, hilar lymphadenopathy is the result of a drug idiosyncrasy. Para-aminosalicylic acid, phenylbutazone and phenytoin are the drugs most commonly implicated. In the case of phenytoin nodes may be massively enlarged ('pseudolymphoma'; Heitzman, 1967).

In this illustration there is no abnormal intrapulmonary shadowing. When present its characteristics will often help to define the cause of the associated lymphadenopathy, e.g. the bilateral predominantly mid-zone shadowing of sarcoidosis, the predominantly upper zone changes of silicosis, a unilateral focal area of consolidation due to the pulmonary component of primary tuberculosis. Metastatic involvement of hilar nodes is often associated with abnormal parenchymal line shadows (Kerley 'A' and 'B' lines) due to lymphatic permeation by tumour. There may also be discrete, nodular intrapulmonary metastases. Patchy, ill-defined areas of consolidation are more suggestive of infection.

References and further reading

HEITZMAN, E. R. (1967) Lymphadenopathy related to anticonvulsant therapy: roentgen findings simulating lymphoma. *Radiology*, **89**, 311
SCADDING, J. G. (1967) *Sarcoidosis*. Eyre and Spottiswoode: London

Answers—Plate 18

18.1 Emphysema.

18.2 'Primary' emphysema due to hereditary alpha-1 antitrypsin deficiency.

Emphysema is defined in morbid anatomical terms as a condition of the lung characterized by increase beyond the normal in size of air spaces distal to the terminal bronchioles, with destructive changes in their walls. The condition is usually classified into 'irregular' (scar emphysema), 'paraseptal', 'centri-acinar' and 'panacinar' types. Direct diagnosis by lung biopsy is inappropriate and the ante-mortem diagnosis of emphysema, therefore, can only be inferred and this must rest upon a combination of clinical, radiographic and functional abnormalities. The condition may be diagnosed at an earlier stage using computed tomography rather than conventional means. Plain radiography is relatively crude and incapable of diagnosing anything less than moderately advanced disease.

Table 4 Radiographic features of widespread panacinar emphysema

1 *Evidence of 'overinflation'*
Increased depth of retrosternal transradiant zone
Low, flat diaphragm
Increased radiographic lung volume

2 *Evidence of alveolar destruction*
Hypertransradiant lung containing few or no vessels, or vessels of reduced calibre, i.e. bullae (when transradiant zone is demarcated by hair-line shadow) or bullous areas (with no clear demarcation)

3 *Cardiovascular changes*
Narrow, vertical heart
Prominence of pulmonary trunk
Enlarged hilar vessels
Attenuation of peripheral vessels

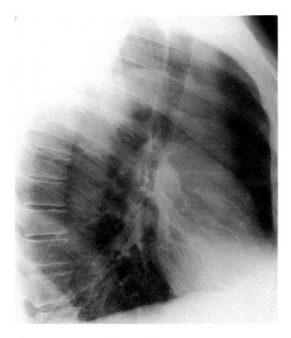

Plate 18c   'Overinflation' due to emphysema: lateral view
radiograph showing large retrosternal transradiant zone, 4.5 cm
deep, at a vertical distance of 3 cm below the sternal joint.

In routine clinical practice, however, plain radiographs
provide useful information and, in conjunction with lung
function tests, afford the best generally available means of
diagnosing emphysema during life.

Table 4 lists the radiographic features of widespread
'panacinar' emphysema. 'Overinflation' is particularly well
illustrated in Plate 18a. The diaphragm is regarded as low in
position when it lies below a point midway between the
anterior ends of the sixth and seventh ribs. It is abnormally flat
when the maximal curvature of the right diaphragmatic dome
is less than 1.5 cm. A large retrosternal air space is illustrated
in Plate 18c. In this lateral film the horizontal distance
between the posterior border of the sternum 3 cm below the
manubrium and the anterior margin of the aorta is greater than
3 cm. The long, narrow mediastinal shadow (Plate 18a) is also
largely the result of overinflation, reflecting the low position of

101

the diaphragm. The radiographic evaluation of total lung capacity (TLC) has been used as a more precise measure of 'overinflation', and the size of the radiological TLC has been related to the severity of emphysema at post-mortem. The method is insensitive however and does not differentiate the 'overinflation' of asthma.

It is generally agreed that a confident radiographic diagnosis of widespread emphysema requires that there is attenuation of pulmonary vessels as well as features of 'overinflation'. Objective changes in the vessels can be appreciated by comparison with vessels in other parts of the lung which are of normal calibre ('marker' vessels). Plates 18a and 18b show contrasting abnormalities with respect to vascular changes. Changes predominating in the lower zones characterize emphysema due to alpha-1 antitrypsin deficiency (Plate 18a). Patients with this disorder tend to suffer an early onset of progressive exertional dyspnoea, usually between the ages of 30 and 45. Symptoms due to emphysema associated with normal serum levels of alpha-1 antitrypsin tend to have a later onset in life and in these patients the disease more commonly shows an upper zone predominance (Plate 18b).

Further reading

HUGH-JONES, P. and WHIMSTER, W. (1978) The etiology and management of disabling emphysema. *American Review of Respiratory Disease*, **117,** 343
SIMON, G., PRIDE, N. B., JONES, N. L. and RAIMONDI, A. C. (1973) Relation between abnormalities in the chest radiograph and changes in pulmonary function in chronic bronchitis and emphysema. *Thorax*, **28,** 15

Answers—Plate 19

19.1 Radiation pneumonitis.

There are areas of confluent consolidation with well defined linear lateral margins affecting the para-mediastinal regions of both lungs. An air bronchogram is clearly seen within the area of abnormal shadowing above the left hilum. These appearances arose four months after completion of a course of megavoltage radiotherapy for small-cell anaplastic lung cancer, the pre-treatment chest film having shown a left hilar mass with collapse of the left upper lobe. The corresponding radiotherapy planning film (Plate 19b), taken supine and not,

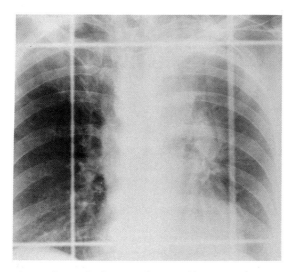

Plate 19*b* Radiotherapy planning film: note close correspondence between rectangular treatment field and area of subsequent radiation pneumonitis.

therefore, directly comparable with the pre-treatment film, nevertheless shows a close correspondence between the size and shape of the rectangular treatment field and the area of subsequent radiation-induced lung injury. The latter's sharp edges, limited by the margins of the radiotherapy treatment port, are a cardinal feature of radiation pneumonitis.

Four phases are recognized in the evolution of radiation induced pneumonitis:

(1) an *immediate phase* characterized by an acute inflammatory reaction occurring within a few days of treatment is usually asymptomatic;

(2) A *latent phase* lasting several weeks follows when pulmonary function remains normal, but changes occur at tissue level – cessation of ciliary function, increase in goblet cells, accumulation of mucus;

(3) an *exudative phase* with desquamation of alveolar lining cells and hyaline membrane formation when the reaction is first recognizable radiologically and commonly referred to as radiation pneumonitis;

(4) a *fibrotic phase* reaching its maximum 12–18 months post-radiotherapy.

103

The earliest radiographic abnormality consists of radiolucency in the irradiated area, but this is difficult to detect. More commonly the earliest recognizable abnormality consists of soft, patchy, ill-defined hazy shadowing. Progressive changes result in confluent consolidation, the limits of which will not usually conform to anatomical boundaries and within which air bronchograms are usually visible. Pleural, interlobar or pericardial effusions may occur, but the appearance of a discrete mass or focal cavitation is suspicious of either recurrent tumour or infection. With the development of fibrosis the radiographic appearances change to more linear streaky shadowing centred upon the irradiated region. Associated shrinkage results in displacement of adjacent structures, e.g. tracheal deviation, hilar retraction, diaphragmatic tenting or elevation.

The clinical recognition of radiation-induced lung injury is of considerable importance, not least because the symptoms and radiographic appearances may mimic infectious processes or tumour recurrence. Typically, symptoms of radiation pneumonitis have an insidious onset, usually 2–6 months following the completion of radiotherapy. In general the earlier the onset of symptoms the more severe or protracted the clinical course. Unproductive cough, an early and characteristic feature, is followed by progressive exertional dyspnoea. Fever and other constitutional symptoms may occur in more severe cases when tachypnoea and central cyanosis may well be apparent. Physical signs in the chest are usually absent. Deaths from respiratory failure have been recorded, but in the majority of cases patients become asymptomatic within a period of months. All nevertheless develop radiological evidence of pulmonary fibrosis which causes few or no symptoms in most, but may cause severe respiratory impairment or culminate in cor pulmonale especially among patients with pre-existing lung disease.

The development and severity of radiation-induced injury are closely related to the radiotherapy dose, the dose rate and the total volume of lung encompassed by the treatment field. Concomitant chemotherapy, previous irradiation and steroid withdrawal have all been considered to increase lung damage. Whereas therapy with corticosteroids may help to relieve the symptoms of radiation pneumonitis, there is no evidence that they prevent the development of fibrosis.

Alternative therapeutic approaches (antibiotics, anticoagulants) have also proved ineffective.

Further reading

GROSS, N. J. (1977) Pulmonary effects of radiation therapy. *Annals of Internal Medicine,* **86,** 81

Answers—Plate 20

20.1 Total anomalous pulmonary venous drainage (monitoring electrodes are present).

20.2 Atrial septal defect.

Total anomalous pulmonary venous drainage (TAPVD) arises when, during embryological development, the normal venous outgrowth from the sinus venosus fails to connect with the lung with the result that pulmonary venous blood drains not into the left atrium, but into some other point of the venous system. Four types are described according to the precise mode of pulmonary venous drainage. In the most common variety of TAPVD (Type I: 60% of cases), the common pulmonary vein has united with the cephalic portion of the left cardinal vein, which then drains via the left innominate and thence the superior vena cava (SVC). This results in the characteristic radiographic appearance of the central mediastinal shadow (Plate 20) due to a dilated venous arch in the superior mediastinum. In 30% of cases pulmonary venous drainage is via the coronary sinus or right atrium (Type II TAPVD). More rarely, pulmonary venous drainage is infra-diaphragmatic via the portal system, ductus venosus or inferior vena cava (Type III TAPVD), or via multiple sites (Type IV TAPVD).

The biconvex opacity located above the heart shadow simulates a mediastinal mass. The appearance has been variously likened to a 'cottage loaf', a 'snowman' and a 'figure of eight'. The right upper border of the shadow is formed by the dilated superior vena cava and the left upper border by the dilated pulmonary venous trunk as it ascends to join the dilated innominate vein and thence the SVC. When pulmonary vascular resistance is normal and venous return to the right atrium is unobstructed there is a large left to right shunt with increased pulmonary arterial blood flow and resulting vascular plethora (Plate 20). Cardiomegaly is invariable and results from a combination of right atrial and right ventricular enlargement. When there is pulmonary arterial hypertension, vascular plethora is not seen and marked cyanosis develops. If there is pulmonary venous obstruction the presentation is usually one of severe pulmonary venous congestion in early infancy.

Long term survival with TAPVD in unoperated patients is only made possible by its inevitable association with an atrial septal defect which allows some of the common venous return to the right atrium to reach the left atrium. Clinical presentation, electrocardiographic and auscultatory findings resemble those due to an isolated atrial septal defect, but the radiographic appearance of TAPVD is distinct. In the case illustrated, that of a 35-year-old male, presentation was with a supraventricular tachycardia. He had been diagnosed during childhood, but subsequently lost to follow up. Early diagnosis during infancy and complete surgical correction with implantation of the common venous channel into the left atrium is now generally undertaken and is associated with excellent long term results.

Further reading

JENSEN, J. B. and BLOUNT, S. G. JR (1971) Total anomalous pulmonary venous return. *American Heart Journal,* **82,** 387

DI EUSIANIO, G., SANDRASAGRA, F. A., DONNELLY, R. J. and HAMILTON, D. I. (1978) Total anomalous pulmonary venous connection (surgical technique, early and late results). *Thorax,* **33,** 275

Answers—Plate 21

21.2 The patient had previously undergone extrapleural plombage.

There are scattered areas of irregular calcification throughout the left lung field in keeping with previous pulmonary tuberculosis. Elevation of the left hemi-diaphragm is due principally to the large amount of swallowed air in the fundus of the stomach. The most striking abnormality consists of multiple rounded translucencies in the left upper and mid zones, surrounded by homogeneous opacification. Several of the translucencies contain fluid levels. While the appearances could be explained by extensive cavitation within an area of consolidation, the perfectly smooth regular outlines of the translucencies and their uniform size should immediately suggest an artefactual cause. Thirty-two years earlier the patient had undergone extrapleural plombage with methyl-methacrylate (lucite) spheres as treatment for left apical tuberculosis.

Before effective antituberculous drugs became available a variety of surgical methods were used to bring about collapse of tuberculous cavities. These included phrenic nerve crush, artificial pneumothorax, artificial pneumoperitoneum, thoracoplasty and plombage. Pneumothorax techniques were frequently complicated by infection or haemorrhage in the air space and were often difficult to maintain over prolonged periods owing to the disappearance of air and the development of pleural adhesions which required repeated section.

Thoracoplasty required multiple stages and, among other major drawbacks, produced marked physical deformity and led to a high incidence of late cardiorespiratory complications. Plombage, a single stage procedure, preserved pulmonary function, gave fewer late complications and became

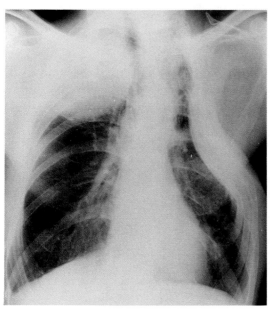

Plate 21b   Radiographic appearance 30 years after right polystan plombage and limited left thoracoplasty

popular during the 1940s and early 1950s as a simpler and less mutilating alternative to thoracoplasty.

The plombage procedure entailed the formation of a subcostal space by stripping the periosteum from the ribs overlying the diseased area. The space was then packed with a filler or plombe. A variety of materials were used for this purpose including polythene packs, sponges or packets of shredded plastic (polystan plombage), lucite spheres, paraffin wax and arachis or olive oil. The exact nature of the plombage material cannot always be determined from the radiographic appearance, although that due to lucite spheres is distinctive. The hollow, transparent spheres – uniformly radiolucent upon insertion – tend to deteriorate over a period of years, some collapsing, others becoming opaque or developing fluid levels. Pressure erosion of the overlying ribs is a common feature of this and other forms of plombage and is well

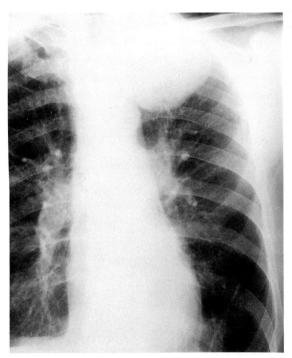

Plate 21c Left apical bronchial carcinoma: note similar radiographic appearance of previous polystan plombage (Plate 21b)

illustrated in Plate 21*a*. The late radiographic appearances of polystan plombage are shown in Plate 21*b*. The smooth, convex lower edge of the homogeneously opaque plombe is typical. The appearance may resemble that due to an apical neoplasm (Plate 21c). In the case illustrated a limited left thoracoplasty has also been carried out.

Although the number of patients still alive with plombage is small, it is important that clinicians remain aware of the possibility of late complications from the procedure and its unusual radiographic appearances which might otherwise give rise to diagnostic confusion. Complications continue to arise in patients operated upon more than 30 years ago. Infection is the most common problem and usually presents as an empyema. Haemorrhage, bronchopleural fistula and extrusion of the plombage material have all been recorded as late complications.

Further reading

SHEPHERD, M. P. (1985) Plombage in the 1980s. *Thorax*, **40,** 328

Answers—Plate 22

22.1 Malignant lymphoma.

22.2 Hodgkin's disease of nodular sclerosis type.

The differential diagnosis of hilar lymphadenopathy has already been covered in Question 17. A bilateral abnormality is the rule in patients with malignant lymphoma which, after sarcoidosis, is the commonest cause of this radiographic appearance. In contrast to sarcoidosis, lymphadenopathy is characteristically asymmetrical and more frequently 'massive' in proportions. The frequency of hilar/mediastinal lymphadenopathy and other intrathoracic manifestations probably differs for Hodgkin's and Non-Hodgkin's lymphomas (*see* below).

Typically, Hodgkin's disease presents with painless lymph node enlargement which may be rapidly progressive, remain static over relatively long periods or, not uncommonly, fluctuate in size. The neck is usually the first-detected site of lymph node involvement. Cervical lymphadenopathy was a presenting feature in 56% of a series of 400 patients (Smithers, 1973). In the same series the hilum or mediastinum was the first-detected site of involvement in 15% of cases, while intrathoracic nodes are involved at some stage in about 30–40% of patients. Mediastinal involvement most frequently affects bilateral paratracheal nodes. Hilar and subcarinal involvement is less common and, when present, is usually associated with mediastinal lymphadenopathy. Occasionally, disease is confined to anterior mediastinal nodes when radiographic changes are best appreciated in the lateral film (retrosternal opacity), which may also show evidence of sternal erosion.

Lymph nodes at any site may be involved by Hodgkin's disease of any histological variety (lymphocyte-predominant, mixed cellularity, nodular sclerosis, lymphocyte-depleted), but a relationship between tumour histology and site of involvement can be discerned. Mediastinal nodes are frequently involved by 'nodular sclerosing' Hodgkin's disease and only rarely by the prognostically more favourable lymphocyte-predominant variety. Large volume mediastinal lymphadenopathy with 'nodular sclerosing' histology is a particularly characteristic presentation in young women. Even in the presence of gross lymphadenopathy, however, symptoms and signs of mediastinal invasion (e.g. phrenic and recurrent laryngeal nerve palsies) or evidence of tracheal or superior vena caval compression are comparatively uncommon.

Pleural effusions complicate Hodgkin's disease in about 10% of patients. Lung parenchymal involvement is common having been reported in 43% of one series of 284 patients (Macdonald, 1977). Two main patterns are seen. In the first and most common variety, pulmonary infiltration is due to direct spread along perivascular and peribronchial lymphatics from enlarged hilar and mediastinal nodes. Such limited lung involvement does not adversely affect the prognosis of patients treated by radical irradiation. Less commonly discrete peripheral lung opacities or, rarely, 'miliary' mottling is seen – patterns of involvement suggesting haematogenous spread, carrying a poorer prognosis and uncontrollable other than by chemotherapy. Right upper zone pulmonary involvement of this latter type is evident in Plate 22. Following successful treatment both pulmonary infiltrates and involved lymph nodes may undergo calcification.

The frequency and pattern of intrathoracic manifestations in Non-Hodgkin's lymphomas are less well documented. In one series pleural effusions were rare among patients with chronic lymphocytic leukaemia, but relatively common (26% of 81 cases) among patients with other Non-Hodgkin's lymphomas. Pulmonary involvement (in 25% of cases) and hilar/ mediastinal lymphadenopathy (in 19% of cases) were encountered less frequently than has generally been reported in Hodgkin's disease (Jenkins et al., 1981).

References

JENKINS, P. F., WARD, M. J., DAVIES, P. and FLETCHER, J. (1981) Non-Hodgkin's lymphoma, chronic lymphatic leukaemia and the lung. British Journal of Diseases of the Chest, **75,** 22

MACDONALD, J. B. (1977) Lung involvement in Hodgkin's disease. Thorax, **32,** 664

SMITHERS, D. (1973) Editor. Hodgkin's disease. Edinburgh: Churchill Livingstone

Answers—Plate 23

23.1 Prominent hilar shadows; increased linear lung markings with bilateral upper zone parallel line shadows; scattered coarse nodular shadowing (right middle and left lower zones); left basal band-like shadow.

23.2 Cystic fibrosis.

23.3 Meconium ileus equivalent.

There are no pathognomonic radiographic features of cystic fibrosis. The earliest changes consist of accentuation of the linear lung markings due to thickening of bronchial walls, producing parallel line shadows. This is usually most apparent in the upper zones. When these are seen in combination with scattered ring shadows (due to dilated bronchi seen end on) and areas of ill-defined patchy or nodular shadowing, the appearances in a child or young adult should suggest cystic fibrosis. Evidence of hyperinflation (e.g. low, flat diaphragm) is more common in children than in adults. Prominent pulmonary arteries reflect pulmonary hypertension and indicate advanced disease. Segmental or lobar collapse due to mucus plugging is not uncommon and, in a small proportion of patients, reflects the development of allergic bronchopulmonary aspergillosis. The radiological differential diagnosis includes tuberculosis, sarcoidosis, pulmonary histiocytosis-X, Kartagener's syndrome, histoplasmosis and other fungal infections.

As a result of earlier diagnosis and improved management, an increasing proportion of children with cystic fibrosis (CF) survive into adult life. In adults even more than in children pulmonary disease dominates the clinical picture and its severity is by far the most important determinant of morbidity and mortality. Nearly all CF children attaining adulthood will already have established pulmonary involvement (Di Sant'Agnese and Davis, 1979). Progressive disease is characterized by a wide spectrum of lung pathology associated with mucus hypersecretion and chronic bronchopulmonary infection: bronchitis, bronchiolitis, pneumonia, mucus plugging, bronchiectasis. Recurrent pneumothorax, severe haemoptysis, allergic bronchopulmonary aspergillosis, respiratory failure and cor pulmonale are all recorded as late complications.

Acute pancreatitis is a rare complication of CF, but is a possible cause of recurrent abdominal pain. Far more commonly this symptom denotes one of the intestinal obstructive syndromes. These occur more frequently in adults (20% of all cases) than in children and in this age group are second in importance only to the pulmonary complications of the disease. Inspissated faecal matter may cause an intussusception (usually ileo-colic) or may by itself produce intestinal obstruction when, in older children and adults, the term meconium ileus equivalent (MIE) is appropriate. The latter syndrome is characterized by intermittent episodes of colicky abdominal pain due to recurrent subacute small bowel obstruction and the presence of palpable abdominal faecal masses, especially in the right iliac fossa. Attacks are often preceded by the abrupt cessation of pancreatic enzyme supplements. The two types of intestinal obstruction can be distinguished apart only by barium enema. This examination may also allow the hydrostatic reduction of an intussuception. Surgery is best avoided in both conditions. N-acetylcysteine given orally and by enema combined with rehydration and nasogastric suction will often relieve intestinal obstruction due to MIE (Hodson et al., 1976). Recurrent symptoms can best be avoided by careful attention to diet and correct use of pancreatic enzyme supplements.

References

DI SANT'AGNESE, P. A. (1979) Cystic fibrosis in adults: 75 cases and a review of 232 cases in the literature. *American Journal of Medicine*, **66**, 121

HODSON, M., MEARNS, M. and BATTEN, J. (1976) Meconium ileus equivalent in adults with cystic fibrosis of pancreas: a report of six cases. *British Medical Journal*, **21**, 790

Further reading

HANLY, J. G. and FITZGERALD, M. X. (1983) Meconium ileus equivalent in older patients with cystic fibrosis. *British Medical Journal*, **286**, 1411

Answers—Plate 24

24.1 Bilateral calcified pleural plaques; right upper zone consolidation containing a cavity with an air/fluid level; partial resection of right fifth rib; healing fracture of right sixth rib laterally.

24.2 Asbestos exposure with primary bronchial carcinoma: the patient had previously undergone surgical resection of a right upper lobe tumour and later presented with haemoptysis due to local recurrence.

Hyaline plaque formation (localized pleural thickening occupying less than four rib interspaces on either side) is a common consequence of asbestos exposure. Calcification usually occurs twenty years or more after exposure and involves the parietal pleura in contrast to pleural calcification following empyema or haemothorax where the visceral pleura is affected. In this example the bilateral distribution of the plaques, their involvement of the central portion of the diaphragmatic pleura and their irregular calcification (sometimes 'holly leaf' in configuration) are also characteristic of asbestos exposure. The use of the term asbestosis applied to this abnormality is incorrect as this refers to asbestos-induced diffuse pulmonary fibrosis, radiographic evidence of which is present in only a minority of patients with plaques.

Typically the plaques are most prominent in the lower halves of the lung fields and are never found at the lung apices or costophrenic angles. The diaphragmatic pleura is usually involved and calcification at this site almost always implies previous asbestos exposure. Other common sites are the posterolateral aspect of the pleura between the seventh and tenth ribs and the paravertebral gutters. Pleural plaques do not cause impairment of lung function and are said not to predispose to malignant change. Early plaques are readily demonstrated in 45° oblique radiographs, while computed tomography is still more sensitive than plain radiography.

Pleural effusions, either unilateral or bilateral, and diffuse pleural thickening constitute the other 'benign' pleural abnormalities associated with asbestos exposure. There is increasing evidence, however, that diffuse pleural thickening, in contrast to pleural plaques, can result in significant impairment of lung function and contribute to disability independently of any associated pulmonary fibrosis and, in this sense, can no longer be regarded as benign.

Malignant mesothelial tumours affecting either the pleura or peritoneum have a well recognized association with asbestos exposure. Mortality studies of asbestos workers have also consistently shown an excess of deaths from primary bronchial carcinoma, the explanation for the right upper-lobe abnormality in the present case. Asbestos exposure alone significantly increases the risk of lung cancer, but this risk is greatly increased by cigarette smoking. The existing evidence points strongly towards a synergistic effect of smoking and asbestos exposure on lung cancer mortality, a finding which has clear implications for asbestos workers.

Further reading

GAENSLER, E. A. and KAPLAN, A. I. (1971) Asbestos pleural effusion. *Annals of Internal Medicine*, **74**, 178

HOURIHANE, D. O'B., LESSOF, L. and RICHARDSON, P. A. (1966) Hyaline and calcified pleural plaques as an index of exposure to asbestos. *British Medical Journal*, **1**, 1069

Answers—Plate 25

25.1 Increase in cardiac transverse diameter; prominence of the left atrial appendage in keeping with left atrial enlargement; distension of upper lobe veins indicating a raised pulmonary venous pressure; interstitial pulmonary oedema with septal (Kerley's 'B') lines well seen at the right base.

Radiological diagnosis – mitral valve disease with a degree of left heart failure.

On a normal postero-anterior erect film perfusion of the lower zones greatly exceeds that of the upper zones because of gravity and the limited right ventricular pressure (about 25 mmHg, systolic). The vessels in the lower zones therefore appear larger than corresponding vessels in the upper zones. Vessels at a corresponding distance from the hilum in the upper and lower zones should be of such a size that the ratio, upper zone vessel:lower zone vessel is 1:3. When the left heart starts to fail the pulmonary venous pressure rises and vaso-constriction occurs in the lower zones. This produces a redistribution of pulmonary blood flow with increased perfusion of the upper zone so that the ratio of upper zone vessel to lower zone vessel may approach 1:1. This mechanism protects against the onset of pulmonary oedema, but results in a raised pulmonary arterial pressure.

If the left heart continues to fail the pulmonary venous pressure and the capillary hydrostatic pressure will rise so that eventually the osmotic pressure of the plasma proteins is overcome. Fluid leaks out of the capillaries initially into the interstitial space of the lung (interstitial oedema) and ultimately into the alveoli (alveolar oedema) if left heart failure deteriorates. The interstitial space in the lung surrounds the bronchi and pulmonary vessels. Interstitial oedema results in perivascular and peribronchial 'cuffing' when the vessels appear less well defined than normal and 'end-on' bronchi appear thick-walled. The interstitial space also surrounds the lymphatics which run in the interlobular septa into the lung from the subpleural plexus. Distention of these interlobular septa with oedema fluid results in the radiological appearance of septal or Kerley's 'B' lines (Plate 25b). Kerley's 'A' lines are sometimes seen as radiating lines in the mid zones running towards the hilum; these are due to oedema fluid distending the connective tissue planes in which the communicating lymphatics run.

In the absence of pulmonary hypertension or other valve lesions the cardiac transverse diameter is normal in 'pure' mitral stenosis (Plate 25c). Mixed mitral valve disease produces a similar appearance when stenosis is the dominant lesion. When there is significant mitral regurgitation there is also left ventricular enlargement (Plate 25a) as suggested by leftwards and inferior displacement of the cardiac apex.

Enlargement of the left atrial appendage deforms the normal contour of the left heart border, which may appear straighter than normal or show a localized bulge immediately below the pulmonary artery. Enlargement of the left atrium itself is usually best appreciated on an over-penetrated postero-anterior film when the right heart border presents a double

115

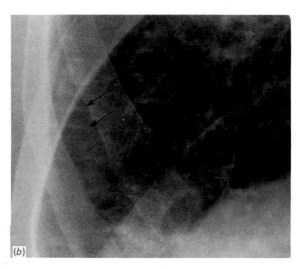

Plate 25*b*   Kerley's 'B' lines: several short parallel horizontal hair line shadows (arrowed) above the costophrenic recess in a patient with mitral stenosis.

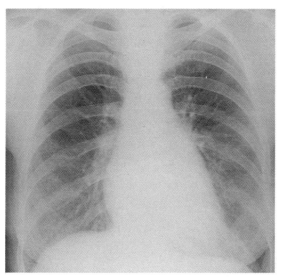

Plate 25*c*   Mitral stenosis: prominent left atrial appendage without generalized cardiac enlargement in a patient with 'pure' valve stenosis.

116

contour. The enlarged left atrium may also cause splaying of the carinal angle (beyond 90°), sometimes with compression of the left main bronchus or, rarely, collapse of the left lower lobe. In the lateral view radiograph left atrial enlargement gives rise to a bulge affecting the upper part of the posterior heart border with posterior displacement of the barium-filled oesophagus.

The degree of left atrial enlargement correlates poorly with the severity of valvular stenosis. A prominent left atrial appendage is usual but not invariable. Such a case is shown in Plate 25d where the raised left atrial pressure is reflected by changes associated with pulmonary venous congestion. There is also prominence of both main pulmonary arteries and dilatation of their central branches reflecting pulmonary arterial hypertension. In about 25% of cases with severe mitral stenosis there is active constriction of pulmonary arterioles and pulmonary vascular resistance may rise to extreme levels. Such cases are characterized not only by proximal pulmonary artery enlargement, but by marked peripheral pruning of the pulmonary arteries, while the features of pulmonary venous congestion tend to become less pronounced.

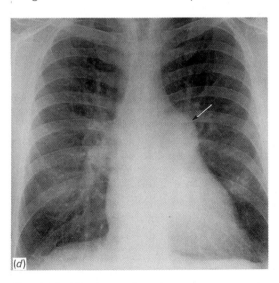

Plate 25d   Mitral stenosis: pulmonary venous and arterial hypertension – dilated upper-lobe veins: prominent pulmonary artery (arrowed); left atrial enlargement inapparent.

Valvular calcification, most accurately seen on echocardiography, is an important sign suggesting a rigid valve unsuitable for closed valvotomy. Calcification in the left atrium is usually located within intra-atrial thrombus, but may also affect the left atrial wall.

Answers—Plate 26

26.1 Right upper lobe collapse.

The shrunken upper lobe produces an area of homogeneous shadowing occupying the apical and infraclavicular regions. Its inferior concave margin is clearly demarcated by the elevated horizontal fissure which separates the collapsed lobe from the aerated middle lobe. There is elevation of the right hilum which is now higher than the left hilum, the reverse of the normal arrangement. Characteristically, the right hilar shadow is smaller than that of the opposite normal lung. The abnormal lateral convexity of the hilum, which in other circumstances might suggest lymphadenopathy, is in fact due to upward retraction of the lower lobe artery and this feature must not be misinterpreted. In this example, upper lobe collapse was due to mucus impaction in a patient with asthma.

As with collapse of other lobes the radiological characteristics of right upper-lobe collapse vary depending upon the duration of bronchial obstruction and the degree of accompanying consolidation. Plate 26 illustrates the most common radiographic appearance. When there is greater consolidation distal to the obstructed bronchus, the area of homogeneous shadowing is larger and there is a lesser degree of displacement of the horizontal fissure. When changes distal to the obstructed bronchus have been slight, the degree of collapse and, therefore, the degree of displacement of the horizontal fissure is correspondingly greater. In the most extreme case the lobe shrinks downwards and medially producing a shadow just above and in front of the hilum, simulating a medistinal tumour. Whereas the unwary may be misled, the associated features of compensatory overinflation, especially the relative sparsity of lung vessels, and the previously described hilar abnormalities will suggest the correct diagnosis.

Answers—Plate 27

27.1 Bilateral apical shadowing; calcification of paraspinal ligaments ('bamboo' spine).

27.2 Ankylosing spondylitis.

Although primarily an articular disease ankylosing spondylitis may involve other organ systems. Iritis, amyloidosis, a variety of neurological syndromes (lumbosacral disc syndrome, spinal fracture, cauda equina syndrome, atlanto-axial subluxation) and cardiac complications (aortic regurgitation, conduction defects, cardiomegaly) have all been recorded.

Lung mechanics may be affected in two ways. Restriction of chest wall movement is present to a variable degree in most patients as a result of disease involvement and fusion of costovertebral joints. More rarely, in approximately 1–2% of patients (Rosenow et al., 1977), a characteristic form of fibrobullous pleuropulmonary involvement is seen affecting predominantly the lung apices. Similar changes are not seen in association with other connective tissue disorders. Early studies had attributed lung involvement in ankylosing spondylitis to coincident pulmonary tuberculosis, but it is now generally accepted as a distinct entity and yet another, if only rare, extra-articular manifestation of the underlying disease.

Pulmonary involvement is nearly always confined to the upper lobes and is associated with apical pleural thickening. In most instances the changes begin in one upper lobe, but eventually become bilateral. In some cases upper lobe fibrosis and apical pleural thickening become extensive, resulting in upward retraction of one or both hilar shadows (see Plate 27a) and the development of bronchiectasis. Characteristically, areas of interstitial fibrosis break down with the formation of bullae and cavities which, not uncommonly, become colonized by *Aspergillus* species with mycetoma formation. Transient pleural effusions and generalized, as opposed to apical, pleural thickening have also been described (Rosenow et al., 1977). The radiographic changes may be indistinguishable from those due to healed pulmonary tuberculosis. Similar appearances may also complicate some forms of extrinsic allergic alveolitis. The aetiology in the present case is disclosed by the lateral view radiograph showing the changes of 'bamboo' spine (due to the combined appearances of

119

syndesmophyte formation and calcification of the anterior longitudinal ligament), which are pathognomonic for ankylosing spondylitis.

The histopathological appearances of the pleuropulmonary lesion are non-specific and the entity is commonly asymptomatic. Associated bronchiectasis or mycetoma formation may lead to productive cough, breathlessness or haemoptysis. Generally, however, neither form of thoracic involvement is associated with significant functional impairment (Gaicad and Hamosh, 1973), because the abnormalities are well compensated by normal diaphragmatic function. Cor pulmonale is therefore a rare complication of ankylosing spondylitis.

References

GAICAD, G. and HAMOSH, P. (1973) The lung in ankylosing spondylitis. American Review of Respiratory Disease, **107**, 286

ROSENOW, E. C. III., STRIMLAN, C. V., MUHM, J. R. and FERGUSON, R. H. (1977) Pleuropulmonary manifestations of ankylosing spondylitis. Mayo Clinic Proceedings, **52**, 641

Answers—Plate 28

28.1 Achalasia of the cardia.

28.2 Pulmonary aspiration leading to pneumonia, lung abscess, bronchiectasis; oesophageal fungal infection – especially candidiasis; oesophagitis; oesophageal carcinoma.

Achalasia is a neuromuscular disorder of the oesophagus associated with degeneration of the myenteric nerve plexus. Defective innervation affecting the body of the oesophagus and the oesophageal cardia leads, respectively, to loss of peristalsis and failure of relaxation of the gastro-oesophageal sphincter. The aetiology of achalasia remains uncertain. The age of onset of the disease is extremely variable, but a peak age incidence is recorded between 30 and 50 years. Typically there is a long history of symptoms predating the patient's clinical presentation. Dysphagia occurs in all patients. Retrosternal chest pain, regurgitation and weight loss all occur commonly, but it is characteristic of the condition that the severity of symptoms varies markedly from patient to patient and at different times in individual patients. In the majority the oesophagus undergoes progressive dilatation with retention and stagnation of food debris which, in turn, results in mucosal inflammation and a variety of pulmonary complications resulting from 'overspill' pneumonitis. Carcinoma of the oesophagus occurs frequently in longstanding achalasia. Its exact incidence is uncertain, but malignancy was recorded in 19% of one series of 24 patients in which complications directly attributable to achalasia accounted for at least half of all deaths (Adams et al., 1961). Most patients fail to achieve their normal life expectancy and, in general, the earlier the onset of symptoms the worse the prognosis. Heller's cardiomyotomy remains the treatment of choice in the earlier stages of the disease.

Marked oesophageal dilatation results in widening of the central mediastinal shadow in the postero-anterior chest radiograph. Typically, the abnormal shadow extends to the right and forms part, or as in Plate 28a, the whole of the right border of the central shadow. The outline of the oesophagus thus forms a continuous, slightly convex curve from the clavicle to the diaphragm. In this gross example the superior mediastinum is also widened to the left. The shadow is often totally homogeneous, but the combination of retained food and air will sometimes give rise to a mottled appearance or an

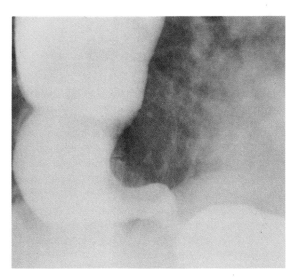

Plate 28b   Achalasia of the cardia: barium study showing markedly dilated oesophagus and symmetrically narrowed gastro-oesophageal junction – 'birdbeak' deformity.

air-fluid level. The postero-anterior chest film may also show changes resulting from 'overspill' pneumonitis. Typically, the gastric air bubble is absent. The right heart border is distinct suggesting that the shadow is posteriorly situated. The dilated oesophagus is often not readily visualized in the plain lateral view radiograph; the presence of a posterior mediastinal 'mass' may be inferred, however, when the retrocardiac transradiant zone appears grey by comparison with the darker retrosternal transradiancy.

These combined radiographic appearances and the presence of oesophageal symptoms will usually suggest the correct diagnosis which is readily confirmed by barium meal examination. Plate 28b shows the characteristic appearance of the lower end of the oesophagus in advanced achalasia. The hugely dilated column of barium ends in a symmetrically narrowed horizontal segment at the gastro-oesophageal junction – the so-called 'birdbeak' deformity.

References

ADAMS, C. W. M., BRAIN, R. H. F., ELLIS, R. G., KRAUNTZE, R. and TROUNCE, J. R. (1961) Achalasia of the cardia. *Guy's Hospital Reports*, **110**, 191

Answers—Plate 29

29.1 Pulmonary sarcoidosis.

There is bilateral hilar enlargement with widespread patchy intrapulmonary shadowing. This consists of linear and nodular elements with a group of ring shadows ('honeycomb' pattern) in the right upper zone. The changes are consistent with pulmonary fibrosis. The patient had presented with skin involvement in the form of plaques and large nodular lesions, which subsequently became 'fixed'. Chronic skin involvement constitutes an adverse prognostic feature, its presence being associated with a greater likelihood that lung changes will progress to fibrosis as in this patient.

Our current understanding of the pathogenesis of pulmonary sarcoidosis suggests that an alveolitis, comprising T-lymphocytes and alveolar macrophages, precedes the development of the non-caseating granulomas that constitute the hallmark of the disease. It is believed that the alveolitis modulates granuloma formation and also determines the progression, in a proportion of patients, to pulmonary fibrosis.

'Pre-fibrotic' sarcoidosis produces a range of radiographic

abnormalities. The widespread shadows may give rise to 'miliary mottling', 'ground glass' shadowing and rounded or irregular nodular shadows. When there is associated bilateral hilar lymphadenopathy (BHL) the appearances are virtually pathognomonic. In the acute stage breathlessness is usually slight or absent and the relative lack of symptomatology contrasts with the extensive radiographic changes. The majority of patients with 'prefibrotic' infiltrates show spontaneous resolution or are left with minimal disease. A substantial minority of patients (20–25%), however, suffer significant irreversible loss of lung function and 5–10% eventually die from the disease. With the development of pulmonary fibrosis BHL, if present, becomes less prominent and may completely resolve. The radiographic shadows tend to become more irregular, predominate in the upper lobes and are often associated with loss of lung volume and upward hilar retraction. With advancing fibrosis disorganization of the lung architecture and the development of secondary infection leads to a mixed physiological abnormality – a combined restrictive and obstructive ventilatory defect. Treatment at this stage is of no avail and progressive effort dyspnoea culminates in death from respiratory infection, respiratory failure or cor pulmonale.

The use of corticosteroid therapy in the earlier stages of the disease before the development of irreversible fibrosis is logical. However, the strong tendency towards spontaneous resolution and the failure of simple parameters (clinical symptoms, radiographic changes, lung function abnormalities) to reliably predict the course of the disease makes the rational use of steroids very difficult. A great deal of recent interest therefore, has centred around investigations that will indicate the intensity of alveolitis as a means of identifying a 'high-risk' group for the development of pulmonary fibrosis. A positive gallium lung scan and a high proportion of T-lymphocytes in broncho-alveolar lavage fluid might help to identify such a group (Keogh et al., 1983).

References and further reading

EDITORIAL (1982) Alveolitis: the key to interstitial lung disorders. Thorax, **37,** 1
KEOGH, B. A., HUNNINGHAKE, G. W., LINE, B. R. and CRYSTAL, R. G. (1983) The alveolitis of pulmonary sarcoidosis. American Review of Respiratory Disease, **128,** 256
SCADDING, J. G. (1967) Sarcoidosis. London: Eyre and Spottiswoode

Answers—Plate 30

30.1 There is a large left emphysematous bulla.

30.2 Factors favouring surgery include the presence of symptoms (breathlessness, recurrent pneumothorax), the relative youth of the patient, the absence of widespread emphysema and a pattern of lung function abnormality that is predominantly 'restrictive' rather than 'obstructive'.

Bullae consist of localized air spaces within the lung parenchyma. They may occur in association with generalized emphysema (see Question 18) or as a result of scarring due to bronchiectasis, tuberculosis or other respiratory infections. The wall of a bulla is composed of connective tissue septa and compressed lung. Radiologically, this gives rise to a fine hair-line shadow, which at least partly demarcates an area of hypertransradiancy. Within this area vascular shadows are either absent or reduced in number and/or calibre.

Bullae constitute the most common cause of acquired thin-walled 'cysts'. Other causes include cavitated neoplasms, primary bronchial carcinoma, lung abscesses, tuberculous cavities and septic pulmonary infarcts. Radiological differentiation between bullae and thin-walled cavities may be difficult when the former are complicated by infection with the development of air-fluid levels. A large bulla may resemble a pneumothorax. In the case of bullae, some lung markings can usually be seen traversing the air space. In general, one should be wary of diagnosing a pneumothorax unless the edge of the lung can be confidently identified, with a clear air space between it and the parietal pleura (see Plate 3a).

Impairment of lung function results when a large, poorly ventilated bulla gives rise to compression of adjacent normal lung tissue and a predominantly 'restrictive' defect. When it causes significant breathlessness, surgical excision of such a large bulla will usually give a good postoperative result especially among younger patients with little or no associated airflow obstruction. Ventilation and perfusion lung scans and computed tomography (CT) scans of the chest will aid pre-operative evaluation. The best surgical results are achieved when scan defects are confined to the area of abnormality visible on the plain radiograph.

When bullae occur in association with generalized emphysema there is physiological evidence of airflow obstruction and impairment of gas transfer. Ventilation and perfusion lung scans and CT scans will usually reveal more widespread evidence of bullous disease than can be appreciated by plain radiography. The indications for bullectomy are less clearly defined among such patients. Recurrent pneumothorax and the presence of giant bullae occupying two-thirds or more of a lung with evidence of compression of potentially functional lung tissue weigh in favour of surgical intervention. In general, however, the results of surgery are poor in this group of patients.

Further reading

MORGAN, M. D. L. and STRICKLAND, B. (1984) Computed tomography in the assessment of bullous lung disease. *British Journal of Diseases of the Chest,* **78,** 10

PRIDE, N. B., HUGH JONES, P., O'BRIEN, E. N. and SMITH, L. A. (1970) Changes in lung function following the surgical treatment of bullous emphysema. *Quarterly Journal of Medicine,* **39,** 49

WESLEY, J. R., MACLEOD, W. M. and MULLARD, K. S. (1972) Evaluation and surgery of bullous emphysema. *Journal of Thoracic and Cardiovascular Surgery,* **63,** 945

Answers—Plate 31

31.1 Increase in cardiac transverse diameter; dilatation of the main pulmonary artery and its proximal branches; pulmonary plethora (pleonaemia).

31.2 A left to right shunt (in this case due to a ventricular septal defect) complicated by severe pulmonary hypertension leading to a ('reversed') right to left shunt: 'Eisenmenger syndrome'.

In cases of congenital heart disease the balance between changes in cardiac size and silhouette, vascular changes affecting the aorta, pulmonary arteries and veins and other changes in the lung fields may yield valuable diagnostic information. When the aorta is large relative to the pulmonary artery this suggests an extracardiac shunt. When the aorta is relatively small an intracardiac shunt is more likely. The combined radiographic appearances may suggest a specific diagnosis (see Question 20) or, at least, a particular type of cardiovascular defect, in this case a septal defect.

Provided that the flow is large enough (pulmonary: systemic blood flow ratio >3:1) left to right shunts produce dilatation of the main pulmonary artery and its branches evenly throughout the lung fields (vascular plethora or pleonaemia). The principal causes are atrial and ventricular septal defects and patent ductus arteriosus. Unless pulmonary hypertension is severe (see below) the distinction between the three entities is usually easy on clinical grounds.

Radiologically, in addition to the aforementioned changes an especially prominent, sometimes 'comma-shaped', right lower-lobe pulmonary artery with right atrial and right ventricular enlargement is characteristic of an atrial septal defect (ASD). Enlargement of the left-sided chambers as in this example favours a ventricular septal defect (VSD) as opposed to an ASD.

The haemodynamic consequences of a VSD depend on the size of the defect and the pulmonary vascular resistance. If the defect is large and the pulmonary vascular resistance is low, a large shunt will develop resulting in an early presentation with pulmonary oedema. If the pulmonary vascular resistance is moderate, the shunt will not be so large, but the patient may still develop cardiac failure at a later stage. The aim of surgery is to prevent irreversible changes in the pulmonary vasculature. Cardiac catheterization is usually performed at the age of two, since such changes do not usually occur before this age. Surgery is recommended if the pulmonary vascular resistance is elevated. VSD is the commonest intracardiac congenital anomaly and accounts for approximately 22% of all congenital heart disease.

The onset of central cyanosis in this non-operated adult was due to the development of the 'Eisenmenger' syndrome, where the pulmonary artery pressure has reached systemic levels. As a result there is 'shunt reversal' with blood flow through the defect from right to left or a 'balanced shunt' with bi-directional flow during different phases of the cardiac cycle. Radiologically, the syndrome is characterized by marked dilatation of the main pulmonary artery and its central branches, as in any left to right shunt, but the peripheral pulmonary arteries become small in all lung zones. Clinically, there is central cyanosis in association with signs of severe pulmonary hypertension. When the syndrome complicates a patent ductus arteriosus there is pathognomonic 'differential cyanosis', the feet appearing more deeply cyanosed than the hands. In the absence of this sign, the clinical diagnosis of the underlying cardiac abnormality may be difficult because the murmur from even a large defect becomes less intense and may disappear altogether as flow across it declines.

The onset of the 'Eisenmenger' syndrome portends a poor prognosis, the average age of death being about 35 years. The outlook is determined by the severity of pulmonary hypertension, and because there is little flow across the defect surgical closure offers no symptomatic or survival benefit and is associated with a high mortality. Death occurs most commonly from haemoptysis, congestive cardiac failure or ill-advised surgery.

Further reading

SUTTON, D. (1980) A Textbook of Radiology and Imaging. Edinburgh: Churchill Livingstone

Answers—Plate 32

32.1 Collapse of the (right) middle lobe.

The postero-anterior chest radiograph shows an area of hazy opacity medially in the right lower zone. The right heart border is indistinct, its silhouette partially obliterated owing to its anatomical contact with the airless middle lobe, another example of the silhouette sign (see Question 12). In the absence of significant accompanying consolidation the postero-anterior chest film may appear almost normal. Slight loss of volume affecting the middle lobe may be suggested by depression of the horizontal fissure. Alternatively, when collapse is almost complete as in the present example the lobe shrinks to a very small size and loss of definition of the right heart border may be the only abnormality. The diagnosis may be easily overlooked on the postero-anterior view unless this subtle abnormality is appreciated, especially since diaphragmatic and hilar displacement are often absent and the altered vessel pattern undetectable. Absence of the horizontal fissure (Plate 32a) contributes to the diagnosis, but is not in itself abnormal as the fissure can only be seen in normals if the X-ray beam travels along the line of the fissure at some point.

The lateral view radiograph (Plate 32b) shows a spindle-shaped homogeneous shadow with its apex at the hilum and its base situated anteriorly behind the sternum. Its upper

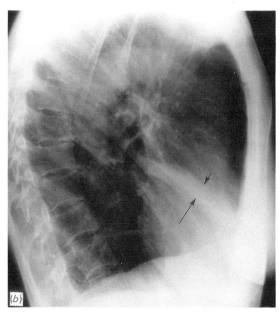

Plate 32*b*   Middle-lobe collapse: lateral view radiograph – wedge shaped density of collapsed lobe bounded by minor (small arrow) and major (large arrow) fissures.

margin (small arrow) is formed by the depressed horizontal fissure and its lower, posterior margin (large arrow) by the oblique fissure which is displaced forwards from its normal position. The degree of approximation of the two fissures indicates the extent of lobar collapse. A lordotic view (Plate 32c) will also outline the collapsed middle lobe, which casts a right lower zone triangular shadow with its apex extending laterally and its base merging with the right heart border.

An interlobar effusion will sometimes produce appearances similar to those of middle lobe collapse. When a middle lobe lesion is suspected, right lateral tomograms best demonstrate the absent middle lobe vessel pattern and are superior to the plain lateral view radiograph or lordotic view for differentiation.

Because it is relatively long and narrow and surrounded by lymph nodes, the middle lobe bronchus is more susceptible than other lobar bronchi to compression by enlarged hilar lymph nodes as in primary tuberculosis for example. In this

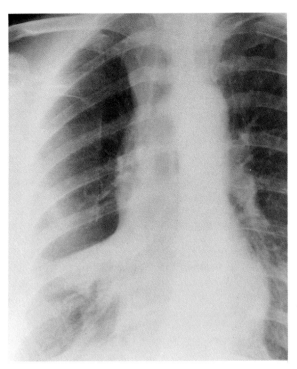

Plate 32c   Middle lobe collapse: lordotic view – triangular shaped shadow of collapsed middle lobe in right lower zone.

case, middle lobe collapse was due to an obstructing bronchial carcinoma. Table 5 summarizes the most important causes of bronchial obstruction, some of which have been referred to in earlier examples of lobar collapse (*see* Questions 1 and 12).

Table 5 Causes of bronchial obstruction

Bronchial carcinoma
Mucus plugging
Inhaled foreign body
Extrinsic compression from hilar lymphadenopathy, e.g. primary tuberculosis
Tuberculous bronchostenosis (Brock's syndrome)
Bronchial adenoma
Other benign intrabronchial tumours
Intrabronchial metastases

Answers—Plate 33

33.1 Diffuse bilateral consolidation showing a 'ground glass' appearance (dense opacities projected over the left apex and dorsal spine represent button artefacts).

33.2 Opportunistic infection, particularly pneumocystis carinii, cytomegalovirus and fungal pneumonia; pneumonitis related to cytotoxic chemotherapy; leukaemic pulmonary infiltration; intrapulmonary haemorrhage; pulmonary oedema.

Pulmonary complications constitute a major cause of morbidity and mortality in patients undergoing cytotoxic chemotherapy for acute leukaemia. The radiographic picture is commonly that of diffuse bilateral pulmonary infiltrates when the differential diagnosis is as set out above. The presenting symptoms of dyspnoea, dry cough and fever frequently with malaise, anorexia and weight loss are common to most of the possible causes. Clinical signs and abnormal lung function (typically a restrictive defect with impaired gas transfer) are similarly unhelpful in determining the nature of the lung lesion. Leukaemic pulmonary infiltration tends to develop in patients whose disease has responded poorly to treatment. Pulmonary haemorrhage is usually associated with severe thrombocytopenia (platelet count $< 10 \times 10^9/l$) and may also be suspected when lung function tests reveal an increased gas transfer coefficient (KCO). The other disorders typically produce a low KCO. Sputum examination and blood cultures will give positive results in less than half of those with infectious complications, while the radiographic abnormality is relatively non-specific. A definite diagnosis, therefore, is often impossible without more invasive investigation. Because of the speed with which death may occur from pulmonary complications, a strong case can be made for empirical management employing broad spectrum antibiotic therapy (including high dose co-trimoxazole and antifungal agents), and possibly platelet transfusions also if the platelet count is less than $10 \times 10^9/l$. Early transtracheal aspiration and transbronchial or open-lung biopsy will provide diagnostic information in 50–70% of patients, but it is unclear whether a more aggressive and invasive policy improves the chances of a successful outcome when compared with empirical management (Wardman and Cooke, 1984).

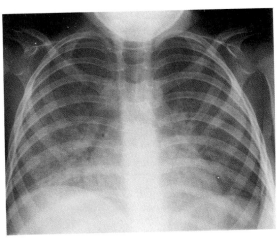

Plate 33*b*   Pneumocystis pneumonia: diffuse bilateral consolidation with air bronchograms

In the present example the pulmonary abnormality was due to pneumocystis carinii pneumonia. Plate 33*a* illustrates the classical radiographic appearances: diffuse bilateral consolidation with relative sparing of the lung apices. The infiltration is commonly perihilar in distribution, often showing a hazy or 'ground glass' quality, and may also spare the lung bases. Pleural effusions and hilar adenopathy are unusual. However, atypical radiographic features are not infrequent and few radiographic findings completely exclude the diagnosis (Doppman and Geelhoed, 1976).

Although it is classically described as an 'interstitial' pneumonia, pneumocystis infection in fact produces alveolar or air space consolidation with a variable interstitial component (lymphoplasmacytic infiltrate). The early radiological appearance is that of a patchy granular or reticulogranular pattern, which is often subtle and easily overlooked. Comparison with previous films may be valuable in detecting early changes. Later there is usually rapid progression to a more diffuse alveolar consolidation often with the appearance of extensive air bronchograms (Plate 33*b*).

References and further reading

COLLIS, C. H. (1980) Lung damage from cytotoxic drugs. *Cancer Chemotherapy and Pharmacology*, **4**, 17

DOPPMAN, J. L. and GEELHOED, G. W. (1976) Atypical radiographic features in pneumocystis carinii pneumonia. *National Cancer Institute Monographs*, **43**, 89

EDITORIAL. (1985) Pneumocystis carinii pneumonia. *Thorax*, **40**, 561

WARDMAN, A. G. and COOKE, N. J. (1984) Pulmonary infiltrates in adult acute leukaemia: empirical treatment or lung biopsy? *Thorax*, **39**, 647

Answers—Plate 34

34.1 Oesophageal hiatus hernia.

34.2 Barium meal examination.

There is a well circumscribed opacity with an air fluid level in the right lower zone partly superimposed upon the right heart border. The lateral view radiograph shows the opacity extending posteriorly from its retrocardiac position in the lower half of the middle mediastinum. The appearance is characteristic of an oesophageal hiatus hernia, the commonest variety of diaphragmatic herniation. Herniation of abdominal contents may also occur anteriorly through the foramen of Morgagni (producing a retrosternal opacity — *see* Question 13), through the posterolateral, pleuroperitoneal foramina of Bochdalek, through congenital defects in the dome of the diaphragm or through a diaphragmatic rupture of traumatic aetiology.

The classical radiographic appearances (Plates 34*a* and 34*b*) are usually easily recognized, but atypical radiographic presentations of diaphragmatic herniation may be a cause of diagnostic difficulty. A large congenital diaphragmatic hernia in which gas-filled bowel occupies virtually the whole of the hemithorax may simulate a pneumothorax. A similar appearance or a hydropneumothorax may also develop following the rare complication of torsion within an oesophageal hernia. Occasionally the hernial sac contains a solid organ (e.g. part of the liver, spleen, kidney) when an air fluid level is not seen. A diagnostic pneumoperitoneum may establish the diagnosis and help to identify the herniated viscus. In the case of oesophageal hiatus hernias, however, barium meal examination is diagnostic, demonstrating the type of hernia ('sliding' or 'rolling') and suggesting the presence or absence of associated abnormalities, viz. mucosal irregularity indicating oesophagitis, oesophageal shortening due to fibrosis and evidence of ulceration or stricture formation. Gastro-oesophageal reflux should be sought with the patient standing, supine and in a stooping position. Respiratory symptoms are rare with oesophageal hiatus hernias unless they are very large. Respiratory embarrassment occurs most commonly following traumatic diaphragmatic rupture or in association with congenital diaphragmatic hernias of the 'Bochdalek' type.

The appearances of the plain radiographs (Plates 34a and 34b), although strongly suggestive of oesophageal hiatus hernia, are not pathognomonic. Similar appearances in the postero-anterior film may result from a pneumopericardium, but the lateral view radiograph readily distinguishes the two conditions. A lower-lobe lung abscess of either infective or neoplastic aetiology may cast a similar shadow, but the diagnosis is usually obvious on clinical grounds. Bronchogenic cysts and lower oesophageal diverticula also enter the radiological differential diagnosis.

Answers—Plate 35

35.1 Pulmonary oedema.

There is an increase in the cardiac transverse diameter and a small right pleural effusion. The most prominent abnormality, however, consists of bilateral perihilar shadowing in 'butterfly' or 'bat's wing' distribution. The appearance is caused by alveolar oedema, the gas space having been replaced by fluid resulting in 'acinar' shadows. These may be scattered throughout the lung or confluent and predominantly perihilar as in the present example where the appearances represent advanced left ventricular failure following acute myocardial infarction. Lesser degrees of left heart failure produce more subtle interstitial abnormalities and other changes affecting the lung vascular markings (see Question 25).

The pathophysiological mechanisms underlying the development of pulmonary oedema are complex. Essentially, however, it may arise in the presence of either normal or increased permeability of the alveolar/capillary membrane, thus delineating two major aetiological groups. Increased vascular/alveolar permeability can be the result of a variety of insults (e.g. trauma, 'shock', drug overdose, infection, toxic inhalation, aspiration of gastric contents, pancreatitis), producing the common clinical picture referred to as 'shock lung' or adult respiratory distress syndrome (ARDS), when intravascular hydrostatic pressure is normal. When the alveolar/capillary membrane permeability is normal, pulmonary oedema is most commonly the result of an abnormal increase in intravascular hydrostatic pressure, e.g. due to left ventricular failure, mitral valve disease, etc. Less commonly 'normal permeability' pulmonary oedema results from a reduced oncotic gradient (e.g. in hypoproteinaemic states) or decreased lymphatic clearance (e.g. in lymphangitis carcinomatosa, lymphangiomyomatosis).

The separation of 'hydrostatic' from 'increased permeability' pulmonary oedema is obviously important as therapeutic requirements differ. In the vast majority of cases, the distinction can be made on clinical grounds. Thus, most cases of ARDS occur against a background of an obvious event known to be associated with the syndrome. Similarly, patients with 'hydrostatic oedema' will usually have a previous medical history of cardiac disease, e.g. ischaemic heart disease, hypertension, rheumatic fever, etc., whilst there will often be leading clinical signs indicating cardiac abnormality or decompensation (e.g. cardiac murmurs, dependent oedema, raised jugular venous pressure, third heart sound, etc.). The radiographic features may also help. Raised pulmonary venous pressure results in upper lobe diversion of blood and radiographically visible dilatation of upper lobe veins (see p.115). Pleural effusions are also a common accompaniment of pulmonary venous hypertension, but are rarely the result of increased vascular permeability other than in the presence of pneumonia, chest trauma or pericarditis. Cardiac size is usually normal when pulmonary oedema results simply from increased vascular permeability. By contrast, cardiomegaly is commonly associated with 'hydrostatic oedema'. However, left ventricular failure may also occur with a normal heart size, particularly when it complicates acute myocardial infarction or restrictive cardiomyopathy. Finally, the chest radiograph may provide evidence of valvar or coronary arterial abnormality (e.g. calcification in oblique or lateral views).

Answers—Plate 36

36.1 There is bilateral patchy consolidation most marked in the upper zones where there are foci of irregular cavitation.

36.2 Pulmonary tuberculosis.

Active tuberculosis in a patient previously infected by the tubercle bacillus is characteristically greater in extent and severity than the initial primary infection. Such 'post-primary' tuberculosis may come about in any one of four ways: progression of the primary lesion; reactivation of the primary lesion; haematogenous spread; or, rarely, exogenous re-infection. It is generally accepted that in younger individuals most cases arise from a progressive primary infection, while in the middle-aged and elderly reactivation of a dormant primary or post-primary lesion is the commonest mechanism.

Physical examination is often uninformative and the diagnosis of pulmonary tuberculosis usually rests on radiological findings and sputum bacteriology. There are no pathognomonic radiographic features, but a bilateral abnormality, predominantly upper zone shadowing, evidence of cavitation and the presence of patchy rather than homogeneous shadowing are all characteristic. The combination of these abnormalities as in Plate 36a is strongly suggestive of extensive post-primary tuberculosis. The diagnosis may also be suggested by the persistence of abnormal shadows with little change over a period of several weeks (other pneumonic infections will usually show significant radiographic resolution during this time) and by the presence of calcification. Histoplasmosis and coccidiodomycosis may cause an identical spectrum of radiographic changes and in endemic areas (North America) both conditions must be included in the radiological differential diagnosis.

The earliest lesion typically consists of a small area of homogeneous consolidation which is almost invariably located in the apical or posterior segments of an upper lobe or in the apical segment of a lower lobe. Bronchogenic spread of infection results in irregular patchy consolidation involving small adjacent subsegments of lung. In more florid cases infection spreads to another lobe affecting the same lung or as in Plate 36a, the opposite lung. The development of thin-walled cavities results from partial obstruction and a valve-action within the draining bronchus. Hilar or paratracheal lymphadenopathy is an unusual feature of post-primary tuberculosis especially among Caucasians, although it is a more frequent occurrence in those of African or Asian origin (cf. primary tuberculosis, Question 8).

135

Longstanding disease results in pulmonary fibrosis and associated linear radiographic shadowing. When there is appreciable fibrotic scarring and shrinkage, there may be secondary distortion or displacement of adjacent structures, viz. trachea, hilar shadows, fissures, mediastinum, diaphragm. Calcification develops over a period of not less than two years. The dense opacities usually show considerable variation in size and shape, some smooth and regular with a circular outline, others quite irregular and having no particular shape (Plate 36b).

While a normal chest X-ray virtually excludes pulmonary tuberculosis, localized tuberculous bronchitis can, rarely, present with a positive sputum in the absence of a radiological abnormality. Occasionally, a small radiographic opacity may be obscured by overlying structures, e.g. an apical lesion obscured by the clavicle and first rib or a small lesion in the apex of a lower lobe obscured by the lung hilum. 'Double reading' of chest films by two independent observers or tomography of a suspicious area will minimize the likelihood of error. Tomography will also demonstrate the presence of cavitation and calcification much more clearly than the plain film and thus aid diagnosis.

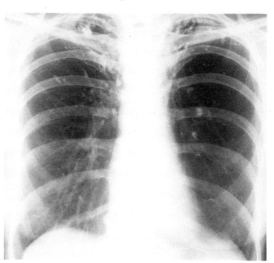

Plate 36b Healed 'post-primary' tuberculosis: scattered irregular calcified opacities at both lung apicies. Note upward hilar retraction associated with upper lobe shrinkage.

Answers—Plate 37

37.1 Left lower lobe bronchiectasis.

37.2 Unexplained recurrent haemoptysis; evaluation of peripheral radiographic opacities; diagnosis of foreign bodies, bronchial fistulae, obliterative bronchiolitis and congenital anomalies of the bronchial tree.

The term 'bronchiectasis' denotes chronic bronchial dilatation. This may be congenital in origin, congenital disorders may predipose to its subsequent development or the condition may be acquired in the absence of any predisposing congenital factors (Table 6). In the acquired form bronchiectasis develops when bronchial obstruction and distal collapse are complicated by infection affecting the collapsed lung segment(s). Chronic inflammation and destructive changes affect acinar as well as bronchial structures. By contrast, in congenital bronchiectasis, bronchial dilatation is associated with dystrophic rather than inflammatory or destructive parenchymal changes. In practice the clinical distinction is usually unimportant although certain congenital disorders may have specific implications for management (e.g. hypogammaglobulinaemia). In general, having diagnosed

Table 6 Causes of bronchiectasis

Congenital	Acquired

1 Congenital bronchiectasis:
Bronchomalacia (Williams-
  Campbell syndrome)
Pulmonary sequestration
Unilateral emphysema (McLeod's
  syndrome)
'Immotile cilia syndrome' (e.g.
  Kartagener's syndrome) and
  other cases of ciliary
  dysfunction (e.g. Young's
  syndrome)
	1 Children:
	Inhaled foreign body
	Primary tuberculosis
	Pneumonia, whooping cough,
	  measles

2 Congenital disorders predisposing
  to bronchiectasis:
Cystic fibrosis
Hypogammaglobulinaemia
	2 Adults:
	Pneumonia
	Pulmonary tuberculosis
	Allergic bronchopulmonary
	  aspergillosis
	Bronchial adenoma
	Disorders associated with
	  extensive pulmonary fibrosis
	  and disorganization of lung
	  architecture
	Chagas' disease

bronchiectasis, the clinicians' role is three-fold: to determine the extent of the disease, to ascertain its functional significance and to plan appropriate therapy.

Although reliable data are not available bronchiectasis is undoubtedly less common than it was 30 years ago, a change largely attributable to the relative success of measles and whooping cough vaccination programmes, and to the prompt and effective antibiotic treatment of childhood lower respiratory tract infections. The condition may cause few or no symptoms. This is often the case, for example, with bronchiectasis following post-primary tuberculous infection when the damaged upper-lobe bronchi are effectively drained by gravity. More widespread disease, and bronchiectasis affecting the lower lobes in particular, is typically associated with retention of bronchial secretions and the two major complications of recurrent or chronic bronchial sepsis and haemoptysis. Bronchial sepsis may be complicated in turn by recurrent pneumonia and rarely by empyema or distant spread of infection leading to 'metastatic' abscesses. Other clinical sequelae include finger clubbing, growth retardation (now uncommon except in cystic fibrosis) and amyloidosis.

Clinical management centres around the application of physiotherapy with postural drainage, bronchodilator therapy and the use of antibiotics which may be required in larger doses and for longer periods than is usual for uncomplicated respiratory infections. Surgery is usually considered only when bronchiectasis is localized and when medical treatment fails adequately to control bronchial sepsis or to prevent functional deterioration, or when recurrent haemoptysis is considered life threatening. For most patients the extent of the disease or poor lung function contraindicates surgery.

Bronchiectasis remains the main indication for bronchography. This still provides the most accurate diagnostic tool and the best means available for determining the anatomical distribution of the disease. The declining prevalence of bronchiectasis, however, together with doubt concerning the efficacy of surgical treatment in most patients has greatly reduced the need for this investigation. The advent of flexible fibreoptic bronchoscopy has further diminished the reliance upon bronchography for the alternative indications cited above. The two techniques can be usefully combined in a single stage procedure when bronchography performed via the fibreoptic bronchoscope may yield additional diagnostic information in about 40% of patients (Flower and Shneerson, 1984). Computed tomography offers a non-invasive and highly specific method of diagnosing bronchiectasis. Its relative lack of sensitivity, however, limits its value in clinical pratice.

In most series of patients with bronchiectasis the left lung, particularly the lower lobe, is more frequently affected than the right. The bronchographic appearances are variable, the bronchial dilatations being either 'tubular', 'fusiform', 'saccular' ('cystic') or a mixture of these. This purely descriptive classification bears no relationship to aetiology, however, and is of little value. The appearance in Plate 37 is characteristic of postinfective bronchiectasis with fairly even dilatation of the lobar and proximal segmental bronchi. Contrast fails to fill bronchi beyond the fifth or sixth generation. This contrasts with the 'proximal bronchiectasis' and normal distal filling that typifies in some cases of allergic bronchopulmonary aspergillosis. When viewed retrospectively the plain chest radiograph shows some changes in the vast majority (93%) of bronchographically proven cases of bronchiectasis. There may be only associated radiographic abnormalities (viz. segmented collapse, localized hypertransradiancy or inflammatory consolidation) or there may be more direct evidence of bronchiectasis in the form of tubular, toothpaste, gloved finger or ring shadows (see Question 10).

References and further reading

FLOWER, C. D. R. and SHNEERSON, J. M. (1984) Bronchography via the fibreoptic bronchoscope. *Thorax*, **39**, 260
Leading article. (1979) Bronchiectasis, congenital and acquired. *British Medical Journal*, **1**, 1380

Answers—Plate 38

38.1 Malignant pleural mesothelioma.

There is gross circumferential lobular thickening of the left pleura. The appearances are typical of malignant mesothelioma (Solomon, 1981) and correspond to the characteristic findings at post-mortem when the pleura is found to be diffusely infiltrated by tumour which extends along interlobar fissures, enveloping and compressing the underlying lung.

Not uncommonly the typical lobular appearance of the tumour is masked by an accompanying pleural effusion, a presenting feature in about 80% of cases. The lobulated

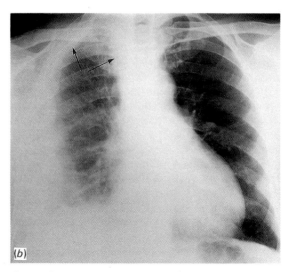

Plate 38b   Malignant mesothlioma: moderate right pleural effusion partially obscuring lobulated tumour margin; thickened apical and mediastinal pleura (arrowed).

tumour margin may be unmasked following pleural aspiration or may be silhouetted following induction of a diagnostic pneumothorax. Alternatively, the characteristic tumour outline may be delineated best of all by computed tomography (CT) with the patient suitably positioned, supine or prone, so as to move fluid away from the affected part of the chest wall. Even when most of the tumour is obscured by pleural fluid the radiological diagnosis might still be suspected from the plain radiograph when there is evidence of diffuse pleural thickening involving the lung apex and mediastinum (Plate 38b). Other radiographic features best appreciated by CT include evidence of chest wall invasion with rib destruction, intercostal soft tissue masses as may occur at the site of pleural aspiration or biopsy, and contraction of the affected hemithorax usually obvious even when pleural involvement is not extensive (Kreel, 1981). The hemithorax becomes fixed and the ribs crowded, with mediastinal shift towards the abnormal side and the development of a scoliosis.

None of these radiographic features are pathognomonic of mesothelioma, but their presence strongly suggests the diagnosis when there is a history of asbestos exposure.

140

Prominent involvement of the posterior and basal surfaces of the pleura and especially of the diaphragmatic pleura typifies mesothelioma. There is no such predilection with lymphoma or metastatic carcinoma, generalized pleural involvement from which may otherwise closely resemble that due to mesothelioma. Accompanying asbestos-related pleural or pulmonary changes in the contralateral hemithorax (nodular or fine fibrotic lung lesions, calcified or non-calcified pleural plaques and pleural thickening) may be noted in about one-third of mesotheliomas (Solomon, 1970) and, if present, lend support to the radiological diagnosis.

There is a close relationship between asbestos exposure and malignant mesothelioma, most tumours developing after a prolonged latent period averaging 40 years after first exposure to asbestos. Males predominate in all series with a sex ratio varying between 2:1 and 5:1. Sixty years is the average age at the time of death. The majority of patients have an insidious onset of symptoms, non-pleuritic chest pain being the most common clinical presentation. An acute presentation with chest pain or dyspnoea occurs in about 5% of cases (Elmes and Simpson, 1976). Frequent pleural aspiration is often necessary initially, but as the disease advances there is progressive obliteration of the pleural cavity and the requirement for repeated drainage diminishes. The clinical course is marked by increasing chest pain and breathlessness as well as other features resulting from local tumour invasion. Autopsy series show that haematogenous metastases are common, but these generally remain clinically silent. Tumour growth along needle tracks is often regarded as characteristic, but is in fact relatively infrequent, having been noted in 11% of one series of 327 patients (Elmes and Simpson, 1976). This potential complication contraindicates neither diagnostic pleural biopsy nor therapeutic pleural aspiration. Significant therapeutic benefit from surgery, radiotherapy and chemotherapy has not been established. The disease is uniformly fatal, patients surviving a median duration of about 12 months from diagnosis.

References

ELMES, P. C. and SIMPSON, M. (1976) The clinical aspects of mesothelioma. *Quarterly Journal of Medicine,* **45,** 427

KREEL, L. (1981) Computed tomography in mesothelioma. *Seminars in Oncology,* **8,** 302

141

SOLOMON, A. (1970) Radiological features of diffuse mesothelioma. *Environmental Research*, **3**, 330

SOLOMON, A. (1981) The radiology of asbestos-related diseases with special reference to diffuse mesothelioma. *Seminars in Oncology*, **8**, 290

Answers—Plate 39

39.1 Intrathoracic goitre.

39.2 Radioisotope thyroid scan.

Intrathoracic goitre enters the differential diagnosis of mass lesions located high in the anterior or posterior mediastinum. The vast majority result from downward expansion of a cervical thyroid, part of which is usually readily palpable in the neck. In most cases the intrathoracic portion is situated anterior to or alongside the trachea, producing a retrosternal mass. In about 10% of cases, when the goitre arises from the posterolateral aspect of the gland, the intrathoracic portion is located posteriorly in the mediastinum either between the trachea and oesophagus or in a retro-oesophageal position (Shapiro *et al.*, 1958). The pathology is usually that of a simple colloid goitre. Toxic changes and features of hyperthyroidism are uncommon. Malignant change occurs more frequently.

The typical patient is in the fifth or sixth decade. The clinical picture is characterized by unproductive cough and an insidious onset and development of exertional dyspnoea due to progressive tracheal compression. Stridor is usually apparent and may develop suddenly when there is bleeding into the goitre. Dysphagia is unusual with the more common anteriorly located intrathoracic goitres and, when present, suggests malignant change. Rarely, as in the case illustrated, venous compression results in the syndrome of superior vena caval (SVC) obstruction. Although far more commonly associated with a malignant aetiology, particularly bronchial carcinoma, benign causes of SVC obstruction including intrathoracic goitre account for a significant minority of cases and because of their potential for cure by surgery early recognition is paramount (Mahajan *et al.*, 1975). Hoarseness due to recurrent laryngeal nerve palsy is also a rare presenting feature, but more commonly arises as a complication of surgery.

Plate 39 shows a more or less symmetrical homogeneous opacity with smooth, well defined lateral borders in the superior mediastinum. Not infrequently the mass is asymmetrical and typically extends more to the right than the left, with tracheal displacement away from the side of maximum shadowing. When the goitre lies anteriorly, as in this example, the upper part of its lateral border is ill defined where it becomes continuous with the soft tissues of the neck. Because the superior extent of the mediastinum is greater behind than in front, the lateral margins of posterior lesions can usually be traced above the clavicle in the postero-anterior view: the 'cervico-thoracic' sign (Felson, 1968). The sign, which is present with the less common posterior mediastinal goitres, is particularly useful as the goitre is often difficult to identify in the lateral view radiograph, although the presence of an anterior lesion can usually be inferred when there is haziness of the retrosternal transradiant area (see Question 2). Lateral view tomograms will demonstrate the margins of the shadow, anterior goitres displacing the trachea posteriorly and vice versa. Calcification occurs in about 25% of intrathoracic goitres, but does not differentiate between benign and malignant lesions.

The radiological differential diagnosis includes tortuosity or aneurysm of the innominate artery, aortic aneurysm and thymic tumours. Confusion with vascular lesions is especially likely when the goitre shows marked asymmetry. Curvilinear or marginal calcification favours a vascular lesion which, like goitres, may also cause tracheal narrowing or displacement. Upward movement of a thyroid mass during swallowing is demonstrable by barium meal examination in over 80% of cases, whereas vascular lesions and other anterior mediastinal masses show no such movement*. The demonstration of radioisotope uptake in a superior mediastinal mass provides valuable confirmatory evidence of a thyroid lesion. However, increased uptake requires the presence of functioning thyroid tissue. In many cases extensive degenerative changes within the goitre result in a negative uptake test which, therefore, cannot be relied upon for exluding a thyroid aetiology.

Surgery is the treatment of choice for all intrathoracic goitres, except possibly when the underlying aetiology is Hashimoto's disease.

* Where doubt remains computed tomography with enhancement or angiography will assist in the differential diagnosis.

References

FELSON, B. (1968) More chest roentgen signs and how to teach them. *Radiology,* **90,** 429

MAHAGAN, V., STRIMLAN, V., VAN ORDSTRAND, H. S. and LOOP, F. D. (1975) Benign superior vena cava syndrome. *Chest,* **68,** 32

SHAPIRO, J. H., JACOBSON, H. G., STERN, W. Z. and POPPEL, M. H. (1958) Posterior mediastinal goitre. *Radiology,* **71,** 79

Answers—Plate 40

40.1 Gross dilatation of the ascending aorta; cardiomegaly; left pleural effusion.

40.2 Dissecting aortic aneurysm.

Aortic dissection develops from an intimal tear which is believed to be the result of either an acquired or congenital weakness of the underlying media. It is generally accepted that acquired medial degeneration results from wear and tear associated with advancing age and particularly with long-standing hypertension. Other acquired causes or associations include syphilitic aortitis, giant-cell arteritis, pregnancy and hypothyroidism. Congenital anomalies associated with an increased risk of aortic dissection include bicuspid aortic valve, floppy mitral valve, Marfan's syndrome and Ehlers-Danlos syndrome.

The clinical presentation is characterized by severe chest pain of sudden onset, frequently with radiation to the back, neck or abdomen, and often accompanied by syncope. There is often a history of one or more previous episodes of pain suggesting that dissection may be a repetitive process in some patients (Vecht et al., 1980). Proximal dissections may result in aortic regurgitation and pulmonary oedema as a result of severe left ventricular failure. Focal neurological signs may occur when extracranial or spinal vessels are involved. Involvement of limb, renal and mesenteric vessels can cause a wide range of manifestations including unequal (diminished, absent or delayed) peripheral pulses, an ischaemic limb, haematuria, oliguria and bowel infarction. The patient appears shocked but the arterial pressure is normal or raised, a useful point of contrast with cardiogenic shock due to acute myocardial infarction. Occasionally, the dissection obliterates a coronary ostium when in the absence of other signs, clinical differentiation from myocardial infarction may be

144

virtually impossible. The distinction is further complicated by the frequency of electrocardiographic abnormalities (>50% of cases) and elevated cardiac enzymes.

The chest radiograph shows a widened mediastinal contour in about two-thirds of dissecting aneurysms and a progressive abnormality on serial films affords good presumptive evidence of the diagnosis. A left pleural effusion is an occasional occurrence (Plate 40a) due to the slow leakage of blood across the outer layer of the dissected aorta. The definitive investigation is aortography when the radiological features vary but include demonstration of the intimal tear, a double aortic lumen, aortic regurgitation or features of arterial occlusion. Computed tomography (CT) provides similar information non-invasively (Plate 40b). The origin of the aneurysm is seldom seen, but its approximate proximal extent can usually be demonstrated. CT findings are accurate in about two-thirds of cases (Goodman and Teplick 1983). It is doubtful, therefore, whether the technique will completely supplant angiography as the investigation of choice. The

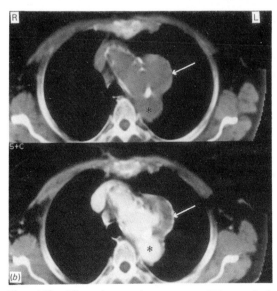

Plate 40b   Dissecting aortic aneurysm: CT scans before (upper) and after (lower) administration of contrast. Dense contrast fills the true lumen of the descending aorta (*). The false lumen (arrowed) is only partially enhanced.

145

diagnostic pitfalls of CT in aortic dissections are the subject of a recent review (Godwin et al., 1982). The main value of CT may lie in the follow-up of patients treated medically and in the postoperative evaluation of surgical repairs.

The outcome and choice of therapy bear a close relationship to the site of the dissection. In 70% of cases the intimal tear is located in the ascending aorta, in 20% of cases in the descending aorta and in 10% of cases in the aortic arch. Proximal dissections carry a high early mortality as a result of retrograde rupture into the pericardium with tamponade, coronary dissection or aortic valve rupture. Dissections involving the ascending aorta, therefore, are best managed surgically. The affected segment is resected and replaced with a prosthetic graft under cardiopulmonary bypass. Dissections not involving the ascending aorta are best managed medically. Hypotensive medication (e.g. infusions of sodium nitroprusside or trimetaphan) is given to maintain the arterial (systolic) pressure at or about 100 mmHg, with a β-blocker to reduce the velocity of left ventricular ejection. Medical management of distal dissections is successful in about 80% of cases. Surgical intervention is required when life-threatening complications supervene or when the dissection is not arrested as evidenced by continuing or recurrent pain, progressive aortic dilatation or the development of a pleural effusion signifiying extravasation of blood.

References

GODWIN, J. D., BREIMAN, R. S. and SPECKMAN, J. M. (1982) Problems and pitfalls in the evaluation of thoracic aortic dissection by computed tomography. Journal of Computer Assisted Tomography, 6, 750

GOODMAN, L. R. and TEPLICK, S. K. (1983) Computed tomography in acute cardiopulmonary diseases. The Radiologic Clinics of North America, 21, 741

VECHT, R. J., BESTERMAN, E. M. M., BROMLEY, L. L., EASTCOTT, H. H. G. and KENYON, J. R. (1980) Acute dissection of the aorta: long-term review and management. Lancet, i, 109

Answers—Plate 41

41.1 Discrete foci of intrapulmonary calcification.

41.2 Previous varicella pneumonia.

Varicella pneumonia is an unusual event in children, but complicates the course of adult chickenpox in about one-third of the cases. The typical skin eruption is followed 2–5 days later by pneumonic symptoms. There is a significant mortality which may be as high as 20%. In the acute stages the chest radiograph shows diffuse nodular infiltration which resolves with clinical recovery. In a small proportion of patients scattered intrapulmonary calcifications appear after an interval of 2–3 years. The lesions are typically 2–3 mm in diameter, tend to be relatively scanty and usually predominate in the lower zones.

A variety of pneumoconioses resulting from inhalation of exogenous particles with high atomic number (e.g. barium producing baritosis, iron producing siderosis, tin producing stannosis) will also produce small but very dense intrapulmonary opacities. In all of these conditions, as with idiopathic

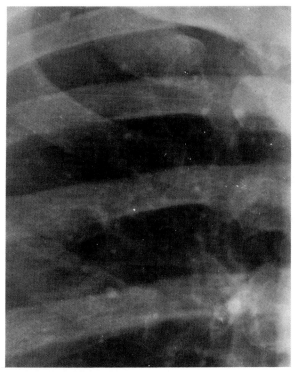

Plate 41b   Healed varicella pneumonia: detail of Plate 41a showing discrete intrapulmonary opacities of calcific density.

147

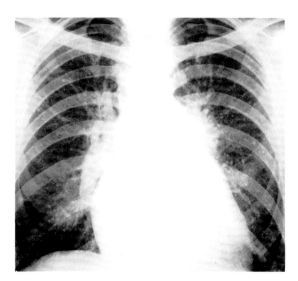

Plate 41c Mitral stenosis: ectopic ossification 2–6 mm diameter, focal dense intrapulmonary shadows (from *Thoracic Medicine* , by courtesy of Dr P. Emerson).

pulmonary haemosiderosis, the shadows are widely disseminated, their distribution uniform and the overall appearances therefore quite unlike those due to scattered intrapulmonary calcifications. Alveolar microlithiasis is a rare cause of fine intrapulmonary calcification with a distinctive radiographic appearance consisting of a generalized, granular, sand-like pattern due to the superimposition of innumerable intra-alveolar deposits of calcium.

The main differential diagnosis in Plate 41a is from healed pulmonary tuberculosis and histoplasmosis. A similar appearance (Plate 41c) is sometimes seen due to scattered foci of pulmonary ossification in patients with mitral stenosis, but this is an unlikely cause in the presence of a normal heart shadow. Typically, the calcific densities in healed tuberculosis (Plate 36b) predominate in the upper lobes and usually show marked variation in size and shape. Similar shadows, which tend to be more uniform in size (1–2 mm diameter) and shape, are seen in the late stage of histoplasmosis (Plate 41d),

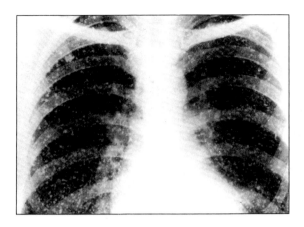

Plate 41*d* Histoplasmosis: healed stage – 2 mm diameter circular shadows of uniform size and calcific density (from *Thoracic Medicine*, by courtesy of Dr P. Emerson).

a condition rarely encountered other than among individuals who have lived in those parts of the USA where the disease is endemic.

Further reading

EDITORIAL (1968) Pulmonary calcification after chicken-pox. *British Medical Journal*, **2**, 68

Answers—Plate 42

42.1 Bilateral apical homogeneous shadowing.

42.2 Cryptogenic pulmonary eosinophilia (synonyms: chronic eosinophilic pneumonia, Carrington's eosinophilic pneumonia).

The term pulmonary eosinophilia is applied to a group of diverse conditions each of which, at one time or another, produces radiographic lung shadows and an accompanying

149

peripheral blood eosinophilia (eosinophils >0.5 × 10⁹/litre).
A largely descriptive classification was proposed by Crofton *et al*. (1952) into 'simple', 'prolonged', 'asthmatic' and 'tropical' forms, with a fifth group where pulmonary eosinophilia was associated with polyarteritis nodosa. It is now known, however, that so-called 'simple' pulmonary eosinophilia (a term used synonymously with Löffler's syndrome – a mild illness, often recurrent but with transient clinical manifestations) has a mixed aetiology including drug hypersensitivity and parasitic infestations especially by intestinal worms. Equally, 'tropical' eosinophilia is not a single entity although most cases of the syndrome occurring in tropical regions are found to be associated with filariasis. Furthermore, greater understanding of 'asthmatic' pulmonary eosinophilia has led to the realization that a majority of cases are related to fungal hypersensitivity. Thus, the various clinical syndromes can be more usefully classified according to aetiology as shown in Table 7.

Among the idiopathic group those cases with no evidence of vasculitis show pulmonary changes of eosinophilic consolidation and form a well-defined group (corresponding to patients with 'prolonged' pulmonary eosinophilia in Crofton's classification) with distinct clinical, radiological and immunological features. Immunologically, the most notable feature is a normal or only slightly raised serum total IgE level

Table 7 Aetiological classification of pulmonary eosinophilia (PE)

1 *Fungal hypersensitivity*
  especially due to *Asp. fumigatus* (80% of all cases of PE in the U.K.),
  Candida albicans – see Question 9
2 *Helminthic infestation*
  e.g. ascariasis, filariasis, schistosomiasis, toxocariasis
3 *Drug hypersensitivity*
  especially nitrofurantoin, PAS, sulphonamides
4 *Idiopathic*
  (a) associated with pulmonary vasculitis (Wegener's granulomatosis,
      Churg-Strauss syndrome)
  (b) associated with systemic vasculitis (polyarteritis nodosa)
  (c) no associated vasculitis: 'cryptogenic PE or chronic eosinophilic
      pneumonia (*see* text)
5 *Miscellaneous*
  e.g. hypereosinophilic syndrome, PE associated with Hodgkin's disease,
  carcinoma

with a disproportionately marked eosinophilia. In contrast, marked proportional increases in IgE levels and blood eosinophil counts characterize parasitic infestation. In allergic aspergillosis, eosinophilia is often relatively mild in relation to a markedly elevated serum IgE. These contrasting immunological features suggest the operation of different aetiological agents and the existence, therefore, of cryptogenic pulmonary eosinophilia (CPE) as a distinct entity.

Most patients with CPE are non-atopic. Systemic manifestations (anaemia, weight loss, fever, night sweats, grossly raised ESR) and respiratory symptoms (cough, dyspnoea) are prominent, with asthmatic features in about half of the cases (Turner-Warwick et al., 1976). The radiographic features are virtually pathognomonic. These include dense areas of non-segmental, homogeneous consolidation with a characteristic predilection for the lung periphery. When the radiographic shadowing is bilateral and extensive, the appearances have been likened to a 'photographic negative' (or reverse appearance) of the 'bat's wing' shadows of pulmonary oedema (Gaensler and Carrington, 1977). An 'axillary' or apical distribution is common and in this instance tuberculosis may be diagnosed in error. Typically, rapid resolution of both symptoms and radiographic abnormalities follows treatment with modest doses of corticosteroids (e.g. prednisolone, 20 mg daily). During clinical relapses there is a striking tendency for pulmonary infiltrates to reappear in precisely the same part of the lung. In most cases radiographic resolution is not associated with evidence of either bronchiectasis or fibrosis. Symptoms and pulmonary infiltrates may recur several years after discontinuation of therapy. The responsiveness to steroids persists, however, and the long term prognosis of cryptogenic pulmonary eosinophilia is good (Pearson and Rosenow, 1978).

References

CROFTON, J. W., LIVINGSTONE, J. L., OSWALD, N. C. et al., (1952) Pulmonary eosinophilia. Thorax, 7, 1

GAENSLER, E. A. and CARRINGTON, C. B. (1977) Peripheral opacities in chronic eosinophilic pneumonia: the photographic negative of pulmonary oedema. American Journal of Roentgenology, 128, 1

PEARSON, D. J. and ROSENOW, E. C. III. (1978) Chronic eosinophilic pneumonia (Carrington's). A follow up study. Mayo Clinic Proceedings, 53, 73

TURNER-WARWICK, M., ASSEM, E. S. K. and LOCKWOOD, M. (1976) Cryptogenic pulmonary eosinophilia. Clinical Allergy, 6, 135

Answers—Plate 43

43.1 'Cannonball' metastases.

43.2 Hydatid cysts; rheumatoid nodules; multiple pulmonary infarcts; multiple pulmonary hamartomas; bilateral mammary implants; Wegener's granulomatosis; chest wall lesions (e.g. neurofibromatosis); lymphoma; fluid-filled bronchiectatic cysts.

Pulmonary manifestations of secondary malignancy are most commonly the result of either blood-borne metastases, lymphatic-borne metastases or direct tumour infiltration (e.g. from a mediastinal tumour). In addition, the transpleural route (e.g. from carcinoma of the breast or from an infra-diaphragmatic tumour such as peritoneal mesothlioma) and the intrabronchial route, as in some cases of broncho-alveolar cell carcinoma, constitute two less common but potential methods of metastatic pulmonary involvement.

Primary tumours from a wide variety of extrathoracic sites commonly metastasize to the lungs. The deposits vary considerably in size from small nodular shadows (1–2 mm diameter) to large 'cannonball' opacities (>2 cm diameter). Multiple bilateral rounded or oval shadows of large diameter as depicted in Plate 43a, especially when they are associated with smaller 5–10 mm opacities in other parts of the lungs, are characteristic of haematogenous metastases. The appearances are only rarely mimicked by benign conditions (see above). In this patient the cause proved to be a metastatic seminoma of testis. Large 'cannonball' metastases may also arise from testicular teratomas, hypernephroma, choriocarcinoma, osteosarcoma, soft tissue sarcomas and tumours of the colon, breast and bladder. Even the largest pulmonary metastases seldom produce a bronchoscopically visible abnormality; bronchial wall tumour deposits usually reflect lymphatic spread. Intrapulmonary metastases, especially from colo-rectal neoplasms, may however extend along the bronchial wall in a polypoid fashion. Rarely, endobronchial tumour deposits may also be conveyed by bronchial arteries and present with bronchial obstruction especially in the case of hypernephroma. Secondary deposits may show central or eccentric cavitation, while those due to primary osteosarcoma (and rarely chondrosarcoma) may show calcification or ossification and are associated with pneumothorax.

Widely disseminated circular shadows somewhat smaller than those referred to above (1–2 cm diameter, small 'cannonball' appearance) are also most commonly due to secondary malignancy. Rarely, similar appearances may be seen in an indolent tuberculous infection, in some fungal infections such as histoplasmosis and in rheumatoid arthritis (due to rheumatoid nodules) and coalworker's pneumoconiosis (due to Caplan's nodules) when the clinical and occupational histories will provide the diagnosis.

Haematogenous metastases may also give rise to widespread small (2–5 mm diameter) nodular shadows resembling miliary tuberculosis. A similar radiographic appearance may result from intra-alveolar spread of a broncho-alveolar cell carcinoma (Plates 43b). The opacities tend to be roughly circular in outline, but with ill-defined margins imparting an overall blotchy appearance to the lungs. The pattern is not specific of any particular type of secondary malignancy, but is

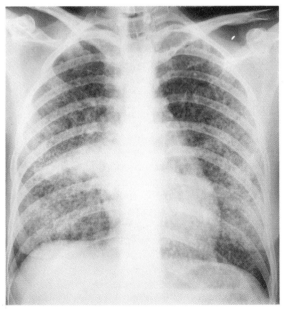

Plate 43b Broncho-alveolar cell carcinoma – postero-anterior film showing widespread bilateral, ill-defined, 2–5 mm, nodular opacities; note also area of homogeneous shadowing projected over right hilum.

153

especially associated with metastatic thyroid carcinoma, and may also be seen with secondary spread from carcinoma of the prostate, stomach, breast and pancreas. The diagnosis may be obvious when there are clinical symptoms or signs of extrapulmonary primary neoplasm. When there are no clinical pointers, transbronchial lung biopsy or percutaneous needle biopsy give a high diagnostic yield. Occasionally, serum tumour markers (e.g. acid phosphatase in prostatic carcinoma, raised levels of α-fetoprotein and the β-subunit of human chorionic gonadotrophin in testicular tumours) will assist identification of the primary neoplasm. The secondary deposits of thyroid carcinoma may be uniquely identifiable by their uptake of radioactive iodine.

Further reading

LIBSHITZ, H. I. and NORTH, L. B. (1982) Pulmonary metastases. *The Radiologic Clinics of North America*, **20**, 437

Answers—Plate 44

44.1 Bilateral pulmonary 'reticulo-nodular' shadowing (most obvious in the left lung field); dilatation of the barium-filled oesophagus.

44.2 Progressive systemic sclerosis.

The radiographic appearance of pulmonary fibrosis is essentially the same whether it complicates the course of a co-existing connective tissue disorder (systemic sclerosis, rheumatoid arthritis, dermatomyositis, systemic lupus erythematosus, chronic active hepatitis, Sjögren's syndrome) or whether it arises in the absence of any known cause (cryptogenic fibrosing alveolitis). The characteristic abnormality consists of a combination of groups of well defined small ring shadows and small irregular nodular shadows – 'reticulo-nodular' shadowing. The radiographic changes tend to be most marked at the lung bases with middle and upper zone involvement as the disease progresses. In advanced cases, where there is considerable destruction of lung architecture, nodular shadows may be inconscpicuous and widespread 'honeycomb' shadowing (due to groups of closely set ring shadows), most marked in the lung periphery, becomes the predominant feature. Spontaneous pneumothorax, a not uncommon feature of advanced disease, results when there is rupture of a small subpleural cyst. Fibrotic contraction of the lung parenchyma leads to progressive reduction in radiographic lung volume as a result of which the mediastinum may appear broadened. Skeletal abnormalities – resorption of the lateral ends of the clavicles and the superior margins of the ribs, sometimes with complete osteolysis of the posterior ends of the ribs – are a less well recognized radiographic manifestation of connective tissue disorders (especially systemic sclerosis, rheumatoid arthritis and dermatomyositis) and are thought to represent vascular involvement in the disease process. They are not a feature of cryptogenic fibrosing alveolitis.

Progressive systemic sclerosis ('scleroderma') is a multisystem disease characterized by varying degrees of inflammation, atrophy and fibrosis in affected organs. The peak age incidence is in the fifth decade. Females are more commonly affected than males in a ratio of 3:1. The major clinical manifestations relate to skin, gastrointestinal, musculoskeletal, pulmonary, cardiac and renal involvement. Survival is closely related to the degree and type of visceral involvement, increasingly adverse effects on prognosis being associated with pulmonary, cardiac and especially renal disease.

Morphological evidence of pulmonary fibrosis is present in 90% of patients. Overt radiographic changes are seen in 25% of patients, while only about 16% of patients have respiratory symptoms, although a far larger proportion will show abnormalities on pulmonary function testing (Wilson et al., 1964). The clinical course of pulmonary involvement is similar in systemic sclerosis, other connective tissue disorders and in cryptogenic fibrosing alveolitis, with about 50% of patients dead within five years. In each clinical category there is an increased death rate from lung cancer which is some ten times that of a control population (Turner-Warwick et al., 1980).

Oesophageal changes invariably constitute the first manifestation of gastro-intestinal involvement and are seen in about 50% of cases (Mahrer et al., 1954). There is oesophageal dilatation with reduced peristalsis and reduction in the lower oesophageal sphincter pressure. The combination of such changes along with evidence of pulmonary fibrosis is virtually diagnostic of systemic sclerosis. Radiographically demonstrated reflux is asymptomatic in up to 50%

155

of patients (Poirer and Rankin, 1972), but oesophagitis may be severe and stricture formation may result. There may be associated pulmonary changes due to 'overspill pneumonitis'. Motility is frequently abnormal throughout the gastro-intestinal tract, but these more widespread abnormalities are frequently asymptomatic. Other gastro-intestinal manifesta-tions include prolonged transit time, colonic saccular diverticulae, and duodenal dilatation with bacterial over-growth and secondary malabsorption.

References

MAHRER, P. R., EVANS, J. A. and STEINBERG, I. (1954) Scleroderma: relation of pulmonary changes to esophageal disease. *Annals of Internal Medicine,* **40,** 92

POIRER, T. J. and RANKIN, G. B. (1972) Gastro-intestinal manifestations of progressive systemic scleroderma based on a review of 364 cases. *American Journal of Roentgenology,* **58,** 30

TURNER-WARWICK, M., LEBOWITZ, M., BURROWS, B. and JOHNSON, A. (1980) Cryptogenic fibrosing alveolitis and lung cancer. *Thorax,* **35,** 496

WILSON, R. J., RODUAN, G. P. and ROBIN, E. D. (1964) An early pulmonary physiologic abnormality in progressive systemic sclerosis. *American Journal of Medicine,* **36,** 361

Answers—Plate 45

45.1 There is a large well defined multilocular mass on the left side of the anterior mediastinum. There is displacement of the trachea and aortic arch posteriorly and to the right. There is no evidence of mediastinal invasion.

45.2 Mediastinal fibrolipoma, thymolipoma, dermoid cyst or other benign tumour.

The patient had presented initially with chest pain and breathlessness. On the basis of this and the appearances of the plain radiograph (Plate 45a) she was erroneously regarded as having cardiac enlargement. Large anterior mediastinal tumours will often mimic cardiomegaly in this way. Clinical information will usually help to identify the cause, but it may also be misleading. The 'hilum overlay sign' (Felson, 1968) offers a simple radiographic means of differentiation. When the heart enlarges it pushes the pulmonary arteries laterally. Anterior mediastinal masses which lie anterior to the pulmonary arteries do not usually cause significant lateral displacement of these vessels and the margin of the mass, therefore, may extend laterally for a considerable distance beyond the hilum. Thus if the hilum lies well within the border of the mediastinal shadow there is little likelihood that the enlarged central opacity represents cardiomegaly. The position of the pulmonary artery may be best demonstrated in a Bucky film or, as in Plate 45c, in a penetrated view radiograph.

The diagnostic value of computed tomography (CT) in relation to mediastinal disease has already been referred to (Questions 2, 7 and 13). In this example, in addition to confirming the site of the lesion, CT has also demonstrated its extent, its detailed structure and its relationships to adjacent structures. The tissue density (attenuation coefficient, CT number – see Question 13) has been estimated for two regions of interest as illustrated in Plate 45d. One part of the mass (region of interest '2') has a negative CT number of −50 consistent with fat, while another part (region of interest '1') shows a water density (CT number +9). The precise nature of the mediastinal mass cannot be determined with certainty, but

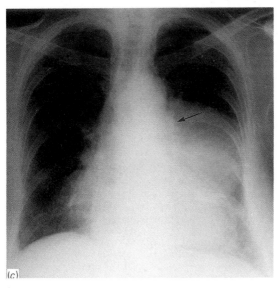

(c)

Plate 45c Anterior mediastinal mass: well penetrated chest film shows the left hilum (arrowed) considerably medial to the left margin of the mediastinal shadow – the 'hilum overlay sign' – favouring a mediastinal mass rather than cardiomegaly.

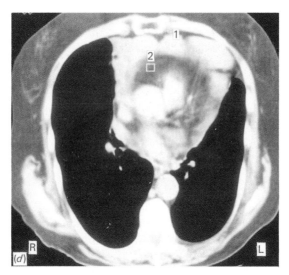

Plate 45*d*   Anterior mediastinal mass: thoracic CT scan at a slightly lower level than in Plate 45*b*; two regions of interest show CT numbers characteristic of fat (region 2) and fluid (region 1) – *see* text.

its multilocular nature and the presence of both fat and fluid suggest only a limited list of diagnoses as indicated above.

Table 8 summarizes the main indications for CT examination of the mediastinum.

Table 8 Indications for CT examination of the mediastinum

1 *Evaluation of equivocal mediastinal abnormalities evident on the plain radiograph*
   e.g. mediastinal widening, prominent mediastinal vessels, excessive mediastinal fat
2 *Evaluation of known mediastinal mass*
   demonstration of site, extent, relationships and attenuation coefficient help to define the nature of the mass
3 *Evaluation of occult mediastinal disease*
   staging of malignant diseases associated with mediastinal lymph node metastases; assessment of 'blind' areas (e.g. retrosternal area, space between diaphragmatic crura, subcarinal region) that are difficult to examine by conventional radiography
4 *Evaluation of vascular lesions*
   diagnosis and follow-up of aortic aneurysms, particularly aortic dissection and assessment of major vessel anomalies

References and further reading

FELSON, B. (1968) More chest roentgen signs and how to teach them. *Radiology*, **90,** 429

KREEL, L. (1978) Computed tomography of the thorax. *Radiologic Clinics of North America*, **16,** 575

PUGATCH, R. D., FALING, L. J., ROBBINS, A. H., *et al*. (1980) CT diagnosis of benign mediastinal abnormalities. *American Journal of Roentgenology*, **134,** 685

Answers—Plate 46

46.1 Diffuse, bilateral, small rounded intrapulmonary opacities. Siderosis.

Parkes (1982) has defined pneumoconiosis as 'the presence of inhaled dust in the lungs and their non-neoplastic reaction to it'. The term encompasses a wide spectrum of clinical disorders which can be conveniently divided into two categories: those due to inhalation of inorganic dusts and those due to organic dusts. Some dusts provoke an inflammatory or granulomatous reaction which may progress to pulmonary fibrosis (e.g. beryllium and various organic dusts in cases of extrinsic allergic alveolitis). Others provoke a fibrotic reaction from the outset (e.g. silica, asbestos, talc, coal dust). In a third group dust is merely retained in the lungs without provoking either inflammation or fibrosis, siderosis (due to the inhalation of metallic iron or iron oxide dust or fumes) being the most commonly encountered example. Others include stannosis (due to inhalation of metallic tin or oxides of tin during smelting processes or bagging of tin ore) and baritosis due to inhalation of barium sulphate during mining or bagging of the dry compound (barytes). Other more rarely encountered non-fibrogenic dusts include emery, antimony, titanium oxide, cement and cerium fluoride. In all cases these relatively inert dusts provoke a local proliferation of reticulin, but not of collagen. Pulmonary fibrosis is not therefore a feature of uncomplicated pneumoconiosis due to these causes. In the absence of co-existing respiratory disease lung function is not impaired and the patient's prognosis is unaffected. Inhalation of pure iron oxide powder (jeweller's rouge), as in silver finishers' lung, results in what is perhaps the purest form of siderotic lung disease. Associated pulmonary fibrosis has not been described. In some cases of

159

siderosis (particularly among haematite miners, fettlers, welders and boiler scalers) pulmonary fibrosis may result however when concomitant exposure to silica or fumes of metallic oxides and silicates produces a 'mixed dust fibrosis'. Table 9 lists the main occupational causes of siderotic lung disease.

Table 9 Main occupational causes of siderosis

1 Boiler scaling (cleaning of coal-fired boilers containing high concentrations of iron, carbon and quartz)
2 Mining of iron ore (haematite, magnetite, limonite)
3 Electric arc and oxyacetaline welding
4 Silver polishing (using iron oxide powder – jeweller's rouge)
5 Fettling (the removal in iron foundaries of burnt-on moulding sand from iron castings using pneumatic hammers)

The diagnosis of siderosis and that of other pneumoconioses rests on the appearances of the chest radiograph in association with a history of relevant occupational exposure. As with all pneumoconioses the radiographic abnormality is classified according to the size and profusion of the abnormal shadows by reference to a set of standard chest radiographs available from the International Labour Office (International Labour Organization, 1980). The radiographic appearances produced by non-fibrogenic dusts are similar in all cases with widespread reticular and small rounded nodular shadows which do not coalesce. The atomic weight of the inhaled material determines the radiodensity of the shadows which are particularly dense in cases of stannosis and baritosis. Cessation of occupational exposure may lead to a gradual improvement in the radiographic abnormality.

Coal worker's pneumoconiosis and silicosis also give rise to small rounded opacities on the chest radiograph. Both conditions, unlike pneumoconioses due to non-fibrogenic dusts, may be distinguished radiographically by their association with progressive massive fibrosis and Caplan's syndrome as well as the upper zone predominance of silicosis. Similar shadows are also seen in extrinsic allergic alveolitis and beryllium disease where there is a tendency to progress to upper lobe fibrosis. Small, widespread but irregular rather than rounded opacities are more typical of asbestosis (see Question 16) and talc pneumoconiosis.

References

INTERNATIONAL LABOUR ORGANIZATION (1980) *International Classification of Radiographs of the Pneumoconioses*. Geneva: ILO

PARKES, W. R. (1982) *Occupational Lung Disorders*. London: Butterworths

Answers—Plate 47

47.1 Left hydropneumothorax with air-fluid levels. Mediastinal emphysema.

47.2 Oesophageal rupture following bouginage for benign stricture.

Perforation of the oesophagus is most commonly iatrogenic in origin, oesophageal dilatation being the single most common cause. Other iatrogenic causes include the diagnostic use of flexible endoscopes and trauma associated with endo-oesophageal tubes (e.g. Celestin, Sengstaken-Blakemore tubes). As a group, non-iatrogenic causes are slighly less numerous and include perforation complicating oesophageal carcinoma, external trauma and barogenic rupture (Boerhaave's syndrome), when a sudden rise in intra-abdominal pressure occurs against a closed glottis. This latter syndrome is most commonly recognized as a complication of vomiting, but may occur in the pregnant mother during childbirth or in the infant during traumatic delivery and rarely also during defaecation, lifting heavy objects and following the sudden accidental discharge of compressed air into the oesophagus.

The clinical presentation varies depending upon the site of perforation. Pain is almost invariable and has an abrupt onset in about 30% of patients. Cervical perforations are commonly associated with subcutaneous emphysema, neck and substernal pain. Upper back and abdominal pain are more usual with thoracic perforations. Cough, dyspnoea, cyanosis, febrile symptoms and a peripheral blood leucocytosis all occur commonly. Sternal tenderness may be elicited and difficulty experienced when passing a nasogastric tube.

The diagnosis is usually obvious when typical symptoms arise in an appropriate clinical setting. The chest radiograph is a valuable diagnostic tool, showing features suggestive of perforation in about 90% of patients. A pleural effusion, usually left sided, is an early feature and is often followed by the development of a hydro- or pyo-pneumothorax. There may be evidence of subcutaneous emphysema, mediastinal widening, mediastinal air-fluid levels or pneumomediastinum as in Plate 47a in which a mediastinal air transradiancy outlines the aortic knuckle. Thoracic manifestations are less common with cervical perforations. In these circumstances, a lateral X-ray of the neck taken in hyper-extension may be of value when there is widening of the retropharyngeal space, straightening of the cervical spine or air in the prevertebral tissue planes (Plate 47b).

Contrast radiographic examination will usually not only confirm the presence and site of perforation, but will also determine whether the leak is confined to the mediastinum or is free into the pleural cavity. The choice of contrast material lies between water-soluble iodinated compounds (e.g. dionosil, aqueous) and barium sulphate suspensions. Barium yields superior diagnostic accuracy because of its greater radiographic density and better mucosal adherence. Dilute

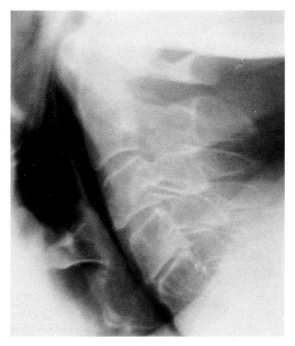

Plate 47b Oesophageal perforation: lateral view of neck showing widening of the retropharyngeal space.

barium suspensions are less irritating to the tracheobronchial tree than iodinated water-soluble compounds, which have been known to precipitate pulmonary oedema. However, spillage of barium may incite a marked foreign body reaction with granuloma formation and the development of pleural or mediastinal fibrosis. This is not seen with iodinated water-soluble contrast media which are rapidly absorbed from the pleura. Diagnostic accuracy is poorer than with barium, however, and as many as 25–50% of thoracic oesophageal perforations may be missed. In general, a water soluble medium should be used as the initial diagnostic agent. If extravasation is not seen and perforation is strongly suspected a barium study is mandatory. Extravasation may be manifested by:

(1) free spillage of contrast material into the pleural cavity;
(2) a pseudodiverticulum caused by a localized cervical leak; or
(3) a narrow tract of contrast parallel and posterior to the oesophagus due to a mucosal laceration.

Further reading

PHILLIPS, L. J. JR and CUNNINGHAM, J. (1984) Non-pulmonary aspects in chest radiology: oesophageal perforation. *The Radiologic Clinics of North America,* **22,** 607

FOLEY, M. J., GHAHREMENI, G. G. and ROGERS, L. F. (1982) Reappraisal of contrast media used to detect upper gastrointestinal perforations. *Radiology,* **144,** 231

Answers—Plate 48

48.1 Multiple bilateral cavitating opacities, some with air fluid levels; left mid zone nodular shadowing and short linear opacities; well-defined rounded opacities of soft tissue density in the right axilla.

48.2 Carcinomatosis.

The most striking abnormality consists of multiple, large diameter ring shadows each comprising a roughly circular or oval transradiant space and an irregular surrounding wall. Moderate or large size ring shadows usually indicate *intrapulmonary* cavitation of which Table 10 lists the most common causes. Rarely, similar appearances may be seen following extrapleural plombage (*see* Question 21).

Table 10 Causes of multiple intrapulmonary cavities

Tuberculosis
Pyogenic (especially staphylococcal) abscesses
Infected emphysematous bullae/cystic bronchiectasis
Pulmonary metastases
Pulmonary infarcts
Hodgkin's disease
Wegener's granulomatosis
Rheumatoid nodules
Ruptured hydatid cysts
Pneumoconiosis (when complicated by tuberculosis or when there is
    breakdown of associated lesions of progressive massive fibrosis)

In this patient widespread pulmonary metastases were secondary to a primary malignant melanoma of the right forearm. Rounded shadows in the right axilla represent metastatic skin and regional lymph node involvement. Similar appearances may be seen in association with metastatic pulmonary cancer from most primary sites, especially with squamous carcinomas of the head and neck and primary neoplasms involving the female genitalia (Dodd and Boyle, 1961). Cavitation may also complicate primary bronchial carcinoma, usually a peripheral tumour of squamous cell type. Secondary malignancy may be suspected radiologically when there are associated small nodular deposits, lytic bone lesions, hilar/mediastinal lymphadenopathy or evidence of lymphangitis carcinomatosa. In Plate 48 lymphatic involvement is suggested by the presence of several 'deep' septal lines (Kerley's A lines) – non-branching, 2–4 cm linear densities radiating from the hilum to the lung periphery – in the left mid zone.

The mechanism underlying cavitation is uncertain. In some instances it relates to tumour necrosis which may develop spontaneously or after successful treatment with chemotherapy. In other cases a ball-valve mechanism may be responsible when tumour erodes into an air-containing structure such as a bronchus or bulla. Neoplastic cavities are typically irregular and thick-walled, features best appreciated in tomograms. Thin-walled lesions may also be seen, however, especially with sarcomas. Fluid levels are considered a rare feature of cavitating metastases and are most commonly seen in association with pyogenic lung abscesses.

Thick-walled cavities are usual when cavitation complicates pulmonary involvement by Hodgkin's disease and Wegener's granulomatosis. Cavitating rheumatoid nodules are often particularly thin-walled and their radiographic appearance may change rapidly. Hydatid cysts normally present as circular homogeneous shadows. Their rupture, however, may produce pathognomonic appearances when air enters the laminated membrane of the cyst resulting in the 'double arch' sign, or when daughter cysts floating inside the primary cyst rise within it producing the so-called 'water-lily' sign.

References

DODD, G. D. and BOYLE, J. J. (1961) Excavating pulmonary metastases. *American Journal of Roentgenology*, **85**, 277

Answers—Plate 49

49.1 Pericardial effusion.

49.2 Echocardiography.

Virtually any cause of acute pericarditis can provoke an exudative reaction and a resulting pericardial effusion. The plain chest radiograph often shows a characteristic appearance and may also reveal changes that suggest the underlying cause (e.g. an intracardiac catheter or pacemaker line, dilated ascending aorta in aortic dissection, changes of interstitial pulmonary fibrosis in association with connective tissue disorders).

Large effusions both increase the size and alter the configuration of the cardiac silhouette. As fluid accumulates there is progressive obliteration of the normal outlines of the left atrial appendage, pulmonary artery and aortic knuckle when, as a result, the heart shadow acquires the classical globular or 'flask-like' configuration. On the erect film the maximum transverse diameter of the cardiac shadow normally lies just above the diaphragm. Recumbency usually results in cephalad movement of fluid and an alteration in the shape of the cardiac silhouette which has its maximum transverse diameter in a higher position than before. This feature may be noted during fluoroscopy when a generalized reduction in cardiac pulsation may also be evident. However, pericardial adhesions as in constrictive pericarditis may prevent the typical postural changes in the cardiac silhouette, while conditions associated with poor left ventricular contraction may also produce a relatively immobile heart shadow and thus mimic the fluoroscopic appearance of pericardial effusion.

A variety of confirmatory diagnostic radiological techniques have been described. Contrast studies may be used to outline the right atrial border with measurement of its separation from the right edge of the cardiac silhouette. Radioisotope techniques have also been used to demonstrate increased separation of the cardiac blood pool from the lungs and liver. However, the diagnostic investigation of choice is echocardiography. In the supine position, pericardial fluid is located posteriorly and gives rise to an echo-free space which persists throughout the cardiac cycle. With large effusions there may be an additional echo-free space anterior to the right ventricular free wall. Cross-sectional echocardiography (Plate 49b) is of greatest value, but the characteristic M-mode appearance (Plate 49c) is also illustrated. A possible error is to mis-diagnose a pericardial effusion in the presence of left pleural fluid. The descending aorta and cystic mediastinal tumours may also give rise to a posterior echo-free space which is more localized, however, than in the case of pericardial fluid.

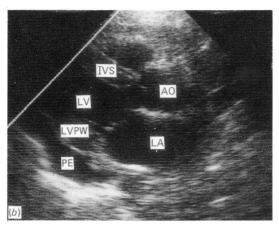

Plate 49b Long axis cross-sectional scan showing aorta (AO), left atrium (LA), interventricular septum (IVS), left ventricle (LV) and pericardial effusion (PE) deep to posterior left ventricular wall (LVPW).

166

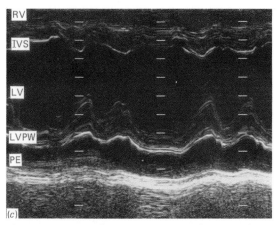

Plate 49c M-mode scan corresponding to Plate 49b showing pericardial effusion (PE) represented by echo-free space deep to posterior left ventricular wall (LVPW).

Pericardial aspiration may be required to provide fluid for diagnostic tests, for the relief of cardiac tamponade (the most common indication) or as a preliminary procedure prior to the instillation of drugs into the pericardial cavity. The subxiphoid approach is generally preferred and should be preceded by ultrasound examination from the same position so as to ensure that fluid is present in this area and not loculated elsewhere. Ultrasonically guided pericardial aspiration using a specially designed transducer has further improved the safety of the procedure (Goldberg and Pollack, 1973). The haemodynamic significance of a pericardial effusion should always be determined from a careful clinical assessment of the patient (Table 11) and management judged accordingly. Echocar-

Table 11 Clinical features of cardiac tamponade

Raised central venous pressure
Rise in venous pressure on inspiration (Kussmaul's signs)
Arterial hypotension, small pulse pressure, oliguria
Tachycardia
Pulsus paradoxus
Dyspnoea – usually mild
Hepatomegaly
Peripheral oedema ⎫
Pleural effusion ⎬ – in chronic cases only
Ascites ⎭

167

diographic signs of tamponade should also be sought, however. These include a cyclical beat-to-beat pendular motion of the heart (associated with ECG changes of 'electrical alternans' i.e. beat-to-beat changes in QRS/T wave morphology), collapse or 'buckling' of the right atrial wall on inspiration, diastolic posterior motion of the anterior right ventricular wall and obliteration of the right ventricular cavity in early diastole; the outflow tract is the part of the right ventricle most prone to collapse in this way.

References and further reading

GOLDBERG, B. B. and POLLACK, H. M. (1973) Ultrasonically guided pericardiocentesis. *American Journal of Cardiology*, **31**, 490

HIPONA, F. A. and PAREDES, S. (1976) The radiology of pericardial disease. *Cardiovascular Clinics*, **7**, 91

Answers—Plate 50

50.1 Diffuse bilateral nodular shadowing.

50.2 Avian protein hypersensitivity (bird fancier's lung, pigeon breeder's disease).

50.3 Arterial blood gas analysis; estimation of serum precipitating antibody to avian antigens; pulmonary function testing with estimation of lung volumes and gas transfer capacity.

Diffuse, uniformly distributed bilateral rounded intrapulmonary opacities (up to 5 mm diameter) may be seen in association with a wide variety of conditions. Scadding (1952) listed 83 separate causes. Variations in the size, profusion and distribution of the shadows may help to narrow the differential diagnosis. Associated radiographic abnormalities (e.g. pleural shadowing in asbestosis, left atrial enlargement when haemosiderosis is secondary to mitral stenosis) may suggest an individual cause, but in general the appearances are relatively non-specific. Frequently, however, accurate interpretation can be made given the clinical context. Thus, for example, a history of malignant disease would strongly suggest a metastatic cause for widespread nodular shadows. Febrile symptoms or constitutional upset favour an infective aetiology, especially miliary tuberculosis or viral pneumonia. A diagnosis of pneumoconiosis is suggested if the history discloses relevant occupational exposure to organic or inorganic dusts. In the example shown, the significance of the tourist's visit to Trafalgar Square might not have been appreciated of the history had failed to reveal the patient's hobby – that of breeding pigeons! The case history serves to emphasize the importance of adequate clinical details, a fact frequently underlined by the reporting radiologist, when interpreting a relatively non-specific radiographic abnormality.

In bird fancier's lung as in other forms of extrinsic allergic alveolitis, the clinical and radiological features vary according to the nature and intensity of exposure to the causative antigen, which, in this case, consists of a serum protein fraction contained in the bird's droppings and also in the waxy coating or 'bloom' covering the bird's feathers. An acute clinical presentation is characteristic of pigeon fanciers whose exposure to antigen tends to be heavy and intermittent. Typically, flu-like symptoms, dry cough and breathlessness develop 4–8 hours following exposure. Clinical signs are inconspicuous, but scattered crackles may be heard over the lung fields. Wheeze is not characteristic, but is present in some patients and reflects an associated 'asthmatic' reaction (see below). Among budgerigar fanciers antigen exposure tends to be less intense and continuous rather than intermittent. An acute presentation is uncommon. Symptoms develop insidiously, patients usually presenting with chronic complaints of cough, progressive breathlessness and weight loss.

Physiological findings depend on the stage of the disease. Slight transient reductions in lung volumes, impairment of gas transfer and arterial hypoxaemia follow acute exposure. With repeated episodes of alveolitis, the development of pulmonary fibrosis is associated with a more severe 'restrictive' defect, which may be only partially reversible following treatment or cessation of exposure. Airflow obstruction may be seen as an additional feature occurring either immediately after exposure and reflecting a type I 'anaphylactic' reaction or at the same time as the delayed 'restrictive' reaction. The timing of this latter response is thought to reflect dependence upon a type III 'Arthus' reaction mediated by precipitating antibody. The presence of serum precipitins to avian antigens thus lends support to the clinical diagnosis, but is an index of exposure and not necessarily of disease. About 40% of asymptomatic pigeon breeders have demonstrable serum antibody (Fink et al., 1972).

The radiographic appearance in Plate 50 is typical of an acute episode of alveolitis due to bird fancier's lung. Similar changes are seen in other forms of extrinsic allergic alveolitis producing acute symptoms. The nodular shadows tend to be widely distributed, up to 2 mm in diameter and, typically, less well defined than the more discrete nodular shadows seen in miliary tuberculosis and histoplasmosis. Occasionally, nodular shadowing against a background haze, patchy clouding and, rarely, massive areas of consolidation may also be seen (Hargreave et al., 1972). With progressive disease nodular shadowing becomes less obvious and patchy clouding, ring shadows and parallel line shadows become more prominent. An important feature of chronic disease is shrinkage involving the upper lobes with upward hilar retraction, when the appearances are similar to those seen in patients with healed tuberculosis and some cases of allergic bronchopulmonary aspergillosis (see Plate 10d). Advanced disease may also be reflected by cardiac enlargement and prominent main pulmonary vessels due to associated pulmonary hypertension.

References

FINK, J. N., SCHLUCTER, D. P., SOSMAN, A. J., et al. (1972) Clinical survey of pigeon breeders. Chest, 62, 277

HARGREAVE, F., HINSON, K. F., REID, L., SIMON, G. and McCARTHY, D. S. (1972) The radiological appearances of allergic alveolitis due to bird sensitivity (bird fancier's lung). Clinical Radiology, 23, 1

Index

Numbers in Roman type (pages 1–62) refer to questions and those in italic (pages 63–170) refer to answers.

171